THE EYE: WINDOW TO BODY AND SOUL

THE EYE: WINDOW TO BODY AND SOUL

An Ophthalmologist's Odyssey

W. A. J. van Heuven, M.D.

COPYRIGHT © 2018 BY W. A. J. VAN HEUVEN, M.D.

LIBRARY OF CONGRESS CONTROL NUMBER:		2018905155
ISBN:	HARDCOVER	978-1-9845-2482-9
	SOFTCOVER	978-1-9845-2481-2
	EBOOK	978-1-9845-2480-5

All rights reserved. No part of this book may be reproduced or transmitted in any form or by any means, electronic or mechanical, including photocopying, recording, or by any information storage and retrieval system, without permission in writing from the copyright owner.

The information, ideas, and suggestions in this book are not intended as a substitute for professional medical advice. Before following any suggestions contained in this book, you should consult your personal physician. Neither the author nor the publisher shall be liable or responsible for any loss or damage allegedly arising as a consequence of your use or application of any information or suggestions in this book.

Any people depicted in stock imagery provided by Getty Images are models, and such images are being used for illustrative purposes only.
Certain stock imagery © Getty Images.

Print information available on the last page.

Rev. date: 08/01/2018

To order additional copies of this book, contact:
Xlibris
1-888-795-4274
www.Xlibris.com
Orders@Xlibris.com
777571

To my father, J. Alexander van Heuven, M.D., my role model and
To my wife, Constance Hay van Heuven, my most supportive critic

The eyes are the window to the soul.

—Old English proverb

CONTENTS

Author's Foreword xi
Introduction: A Word about Ophthalmology xiii

PART I

EARLY LESSONS

Chapter 1: Early Signs 3
Chapter 2: The Complete Eye Exam 7
Chapter 3: The Teacher 12
Chapter 4: Look and You Shall Find 16
Chapter 5: The Learning Process 23
Chapter 6: Can You See? 26
      A. Suzan 26
      B. Antonio 28
      C. Alexandra 31
      D. Joe 33
      E. Veronica 36
Chapter 7: A New Disease 40

PART II

TOO MUCH FOCUS

Chapter 1: The Second Eye 49
Chapter 2: Routines 54
Chapter 3: Is this Research or What? 59

Part III

Keep Your Eyes Open

Chapter 1: The Fiancé 67
Chapter 2: The Turtleneck 73
Chapter 3: White Spots 79
Chapter 4: Deviation 86
Chapter 5: Black Spots 97

Part IV

Listen and You Will See

Chapter 1: New Knowledge 107
Chapter 2: Insult 114
Chapter 3: Playing God 120
Chapter 4: Chief Complaint 126
Chapter 5: The Patient Knows Best 133

Part V

Adjustments

Chapter 1: Unrealized Potential 141
Chapter 2: Children 147
Chapter 3: Judgment 151
Chapter 4: Mamma Mia 159

Part VI

Are They Crazy?

Chapter 1: Afraid 163
Chapter 2: Give Me a Break 170

Part VII

The Doctor Perseveres

Chapter 1: The Graduate 179
Chapter 2: Iron Lady 186
Chapter 3: Elite 193

Part VIII

Divine Intervention

Chapter 1: Salvation 205
Chapter 2: The Power of the Church 212
Chapter 3: Oops 220

Part IX

The Ophthalmologist as a Hero

Chapter 1: She Gave What She Could 227
Chapter 2: Growing Up Fast 233
Chapter 3: I'll Forever Love You 243
Chapter 4: Dependence 251
Chapter 5: Pallbearer 258

Author's Foreword

The most feared loss of function during life is the loss of sight. Thus, the prevention of blindness is of the greatest importance to humankind. This is the task of the ophthalmologist and is the subject of this book.

These chapters are a series of true stories about actual patients I saw during my six years of ophthalmic training and a subsequent fifty years of academic medical school practice at several universities. The few dozen patients I describe were especially memorable because they were interesting people, with interesting problems, that provided me with many teachable moments that occur in an ophthalmic practice. I have already told these stories in multiple classrooms and professional meetings to a variety of audiences including medical students, residents, and colleagues. I am now telling them to a larger audience. I have also included some stories told to me by my father, also an academic ophthalmologist first at the University of Utrecht in the Netherlands and later at Yale University. His interests in the combination of scientific research, teaching, and patient care were an example I could hardly ignore and helped stimulate me to follow in his footsteps. I also remember the patients' elation I witnessed at age seven or eight when, on some Saturdays, I accompanied my father on his postcataract rounds, removing the bandage for the first time from an eye that had been blind the day before and could now see. Later, when I was ten or eleven, I was permitted to watch eye surgeries and even occasionally assist. Then there were weekends when my father and I would go to the basement and practice doing corneal transplants on pig eyes from the slaughterhouse.

Clearly, with such a background, how could I not have become an ophthalmologist?

From the index of chapter headings, it is easy to see a great variety of topics, including how doctors learn from their teachers and also from their patients. There are also stories about learning to interact with patients to gain their confidence. Other chapters emphasize observing, attention to detail, listening, and understanding the patient's true concerns, such as the fear of going blind.

Since everything described in this book actually happened, it was important to assure patient confidentiality. Thus, in each case, the name and physical description of the patient has been changed, as well as the circumstances surrounding the case. Often, two or three patients with similar stories have been coalesced into a single patient. As a result, individual patients are really impossible to recognize. However, I personally remember each of them well and thank them all for giving me great memories. They made my life as a teacher easier and, as an academician, more fulfilling.

Introduction

A WORD ABOUT OPHTHALMOLOGY

Ophthalmology is classified as a surgical subspecialty. However, it is largely nonsurgical and deals mostly with medically treated eye conditions as well as many systemic diseases, which are often visible in the eye long before they cause general signs or symptoms. This is famously true, for example, in adult onset diabetes, where the diagnosis in over 60 percent is first made by the ophthalmologist, according to a decade-old study from Great Britain.

The reason why an eye MD can often make early diagnoses stems from the unique structure of the eye, which combines transparency with an optical system that focuses light. Thus, the examiner can truly get a clear picture of the inside of the organ and see blood vessels, nerves, blood cells, and pathologic deposits, which help the physician narrow the differential diagnostic list even before a single blood test is done. Unlike many fields in modern medicine, where laboratory tests and imaging studies are often ordered before the doctor even touches the patient, ophthalmologists still rely heavily on the art of physical diagnosis. They know that many common diseases, such as syphilis, tuberculosis, AIDS, rheumatoid arthritis, some fungal and parasitic diseases, immunological disorders, and many others, have specific footprints visible within the eye. Because of this, eye doctors, family practitioners, pediatricians, and internists are in constant dialogue with one another and rely heavily on one another as well.

In addition, primary care providers and ophthalmologists have something else in common. They both get to know their patients very well, sometimes even for a lifetime, which makes their practice of medicine more interesting and rewarding.

Part I

Early Lessons

Chapter 1: Early Signs 3
Chapter 2: The Complete Eye Exam 7
Chapter 3: The Teacher 12
Chapter 4: Look and You Shall Find 16
Chapter 5: The Learning Process..23
Chapter 6: Can You See? 26
     A. Suzan 26
     B. Antonio 28
     C. Alexandra 31
     D. Joe 33
     E. Veronica 36
Chapter 7: A New Disease 40

Chapter 1

EARLY SIGNS

It's hard to keep children out of the poison ivy. The New England shore is full of it—at the edge of many beach paths, on that little slope where the sand is piled up. "Watch out for the three-leaf pattern!" How many times have we said it?

Having returned from Nantucket six weeks before, the six-year-old boy being brought in by his mother was obviously unhappy and rather subdued. The mother, on the other hand, seemed a bit frantic. "This started about two months ago. I had told him to stay away from the poison ivy. We showed him what it looked like. He was so good in the beginning of the summer. All the other kids got it right away, but not Joey." Turning her head to look at the boy, she said, "Why did you do this now, when it was almost time to go home and go back to school? I thought you liked school." The child said nothing and looked down at the floor from the edge of the chair.

"Does it still itch?" I asked. He nodded no but still remained quiet. "Let me see what you look like." I raised the electric exam chair and shone my little penlight on his bare arms and hands. "It's mostly on his face now," said the mother, "but it started all over his arms, especially his right arm, and his legs too. It seemed like he kept getting into the poison ivy over and over again—first with his face, with redness around his eye. Then his arms, they really itched.

W. A. J. VAN HEUVEN, M.D.

I treated that with some anti-itch ointment I had. Then his arms and one leg became all blisters, so I took him to the Nantucket Hospital emergency room. They said it was poison ivy. They said he was lucky not to get the blisters on his face and inside his eye. They also explained that it could have just been one exposure to different amounts of the toxin, or else multiple exposures, to explain why it wasn't all at the same stage in different places of his body. In any case, they told me to continue the anti-itch ointment, which seemed to help, and also gave me some calamine lotion to help soothe the affected areas, which might stop Joey from scratching. As far as the blisters were concerned, the doctor gave me some other stuff. I think it was Bert's or, or, or, no . . . Burrow's solution to dry things up before applying the other ointments. He also told me to wash his beach towel and even to give our dog a bath to get rid of any poison ivy toxin, which might kept reinfecting Joey. In any case, he assured us that the blisters were not contagious, even though all the other kids and their parents were sure that they were. It really put a damper on the last few weeks of the summer. Our neighbors wouldn't let Joey play with their three children, thinking they would get it too. They had already had it in June."

The child's arms and legs (he was wearing shorts and sandals) looked pretty normal to me. Knowing the story, I could detect some scaling on both arms and felt some roughness, but nothing that would make the diagnosis of poison ivy at this stage. I lifted the child's chin with my right hand and could see that the area around his left eye was red and possibly a little swollen, especially the upper lid, which was drooping halfway across his pupil. "Can you open your eyes wide?" I asked. He tried, but the lid remained droopy. Turning to the mother on my left, I asked, "Has he had a droopy lid all along?"

"Well," she said, "the poison ivy really started around his left eye. Maybe it was a little droopy from the start, but then the redness increased, and Joey said that he saw double. So we went to see the visiting eye doctor on the island, who comes once every two weeks, and he mentioned cellulitis." She fiddled in her pocketbook and pulled out a slip of yellow paper. "Here, I wrote it down. So he gave me a prescription for penicillin, which Joey took for seven days, four times a day. It made him feel sick." She nodded toward the child to get him to agree. "And it didn't even help. The redness just stayed. His lid was droopy, but it didn't seem to hurt or bother him except for his complaint of double vision at times, not like how the blisters bothered him. That was the worst of it—itching, scratching, blisters—all that lotion and goo that we used. What a mess!"

When I lifted up the lid, it was the first time the child spoke. "I see double. Now I see double." I covered one eye and then the other, and it became clear that the eyes were not aligned. The left eye seemed to be pushed down. As I tested the eye movements, it also showed that the eye motion was restricted, especially looking down. Using an exophthalmometer, the left eye was more prominent and was pushed forward about three millimeters.

The examination did not seem to hurt the child. As I completed it, I found nothing else. The vision was good, the eye pressure was normal, and the retina and optic nerve, which I could see after dilating the pupil with drops, were both normal. Because of the absence of any signs of infection or inflammation at this point, I told the mother that we needed to do some tests to see what was causing the eye to be so swollen. This being 1963, none of today's tests, such as MRI, existed, but I ordered more blood tests, including thyroid tests, and scheduled an x-ray and an orbital ultrasound. Three days later, when I had the results, I saw the child again. By now, the bulging forward of the eye was four millimeters at least. The blood tests were normal, but the ultrasound demonstrated a possible tumor behind the left eye. A biopsy was scheduled the following Monday in the operating room. That Thursday, the pathologist reported an embryonal rhabdomyosarcoma of the eye muscles, the most aggressive form of this type of muscle cancer known. It was devastating news and a total surprise to the family.

Subsequently, after long discussions, the parents agreed on an exenteration of the left orbit, even though the prognosis was grim. The operation removed all the contents of the orbit, including the eyelids, so that eventually, plastic surgery with some sort of facial implant would have to be done for cosmesis. Two months later, the child became ill with brain and other metastases. Chemotherapy was in its infancy, and radiation treatment was never done. The child had had enough! Within three months, he died, only six months after the first redness around the eye appeared. "Why did I not take him right away to an ophthalmologist?" the mother chided herself. Why did no one, not even the doctors, see that the eye problem was different from the poison ivy—no itching and no blisters? Would earlier detection not have saved his life? It was difficult for me to tell the parents that it might not have made any difference in 1963, because this highly malignant cancer resulted in a near 100 percent death rate within a year.

Fortunately today, this is no longer true, due to the development of immunotherapy, chemotherapy, and focal radiation methods. Today, the survival rate approaches 70 percent, and early detection clearly makes a difference. However, I ask, are we more observant today to assure early detection?

Chapter 2

THE COMPLETE EYE EXAM

Ophthalmology is the only surgical subspecialty where a complete eye examination is done routinely on most patients on a regular basis. It is thought that no matter what the patient's chief complaint may be, such an exam uncovers most eye conditions of any significance. Ophthalmology thus continues to be a specialty where physical diagnosis is the key to a cure. This is now very different from most other areas of medicine, where laboratory tests are substituted for a physical examination in large part.

This concept of a complete eye examination must be taught, because it is easy for any ophthalmologist to forget to do that when a chief complaint by a patient can be easily diagnosed or treated simply by a focused and quick evaluation. Itchy red eyes mean allergic conjunctivitis, and the treatment is some mast-cell stabilizing eye drops. Blurry vision while reading in a forty-year-old means presbyopia, and reading glasses are needed. The list goes on.

Joy, a sixteen-year-old patient, a contact lens wearer, came to the office with a very red eye and lid swelling on the left side. The optometrist, who had prescribed the lenses, gave her a combination eye drop that contained an antibiotic and a steroid (cortisone). This is usually what nonophthalmologists do, because it treats both the infection and the inflammation, no matter what the diagnosis might be, and it often works. Notwithstanding the high success rate, it does not address the cause of the problem. It is similar to giving aspirin for a persistent headache. Who knows what is causing it? Especially if it is chronic and severe, could it be that rare brain tumor? Probably not, and aspirin works.

During the first day of treatment, the patient reported an improvement in the symptoms. She had returned to the eye doctor, and he had continued the same regimen: two drops in the left eye four times daily. Then the improvement ceased, and on the third day, he examined her again. The upper eyelid was still swollen, and some yellow purulent discharge (pus) was still coating the eyelashes. Now he looked at her more closely. Pulling her lower lid down and then her upper lid upward to expose the conjunctiva, he could see that it was inflamed, especially above. No source of the problem could be found. However, the girl reported that it hurt when he touched her upper lid. He looked for some foreign body, some speck of dirt or dust, but saw none. He used the slit lamp's magnification to look at the eye surface, the cornea. Using a drop of fluorescein stain and examining under a blue light, the surface appeared normal—no staining. He was pleased that there was no corneal ulcer, which would have been serious, although quite common in contact lens patients, especially teenagers whose daily life was often erratic enough to be incompatible with following a prescribed protocol for safe contact lens wear. Also, cortisone eye drops, which decreased nonspecific inflammation but promoted bacterial or fungal infection, would be contraindicated. He decided to change the eye drops and now prescribed a more broad-spectrum antibiotic and also Pred Forte, a potent cortisone drop, to be taken six times a day. He also, again, emphasized that she should not wear her contacts while she had this problem.

"I can't anyway" was the answer. "I lost the lens."

When the redness, discharge, and discomfort continued unabatedly for another three days, the optometrist was tempted to send the patient to the local hospital laboratory for an analysis of the purulent discharge—a culture and sensitivity test, which might pinpoint the organism causing the infection—but he really did not feel comfortable dealing with all that information, which was also clearly outside his area of expertise. And so he referred the patient to a medical eye doctor.

The ophthalmologist, a young man with an Indian accent, was kind and polite and seemed very thorough. He also determined that the problem was not with the eye itself. The vision was good, the pupils reacted normally to light, eye movements were good in all directions but felt slightly painful looking up, and the cornea did not stain with fluorescein. There was no sign of intraocular inflammation. He, too, looked for a foreign body. Pulling down the lower lid while the girl looked up, squirming slightly, he saw nothing abnormal. Then, with the patient looking down, he pressed on the upper lid with a cotton-tipped applicator and was able to flip or evert the upper eyelid, where small foreign bodies frequently lodge. He saw nothing but a glob of yellow pus emerging. He wiped that away with another Q-tip, which he placed into a tube of blood agar to be sent to the lab for a diagnostic culture. He also smeared some pus on a glass slide that he would send to be stained and viewed under a microscope. The result of the microscopic exam would be available the next day and might just identify the infecting organism. The result of the culture would take three days but would also tell him which antibiotic would most likely cure the infection. He told Joy to stop the cortisone drops until he knew more from the cultures. "By the way, use some hot soaks also. Three times a day, get a washcloth dipped in hot water and hold it on your eye for five minutes. Keep it hot, but don't burn yourself. I'll call you when I have the results of the culture tests."

Late in the afternoon, two days later, he called Joy on her cell phone. "Are you better?" He wanted to know.

"No, not really," she replied.

"Any more pain?"

"About the same, and I still have that goo coming out of my eye. I'm putting in the drops, and I'm doing the soaks. My boyfriend is afraid that he's going to catch it."

"Well, the cultures showed that we are using correct antibiotic drops, so keep up whatever you are doing and let us see you in a couple of days."

The following day, Joy's high school teacher called her mother. She, too, thought that Joy's red eye might be contagious and wondered if Joy should continue coming to class. The conversation led to a decision to get another opinion. The mother called around to several of her closest friends for a suggestion about the best place to go. Finally, someone suggested that she should go to Boston, which was only forty miles away.

"Certainly, they should have good doctors at the Massachusetts Eye and Ear Infirmary. They even have an eye emergency room over there. You can just go. You don't even need an appointment."

Joy and her mother went together.

The resident was a very tall young-looking boy with red hair and freckles. It was hard to believe that he was more than eighteen years old. He took an extensive history. He wanted to know everything about Joy's health. Then he zeroed in on her contact lens loss. How did she lose it? Had she ever lost one before? What did she usually do to find a lost lens?

"Well, sometimes the lens gets displaced upwards. It is still on my eye, but not on my cornea. If I look way down, I can sometimes get it down with my finger from where it is stuck under my upper lid. My mom sometimes can see it up there and helps me get it out."

The resident then proceeded with the same familiar eye exam Joy had had before. Again, the eye itself was found to be normal. He now placed some anesthetic eye drops in the eye and warned her he was going to flip her upper lid. More pus came out, which he wiped away. He asked one of the technicians to help him. "I think she has a contact lens stuck way up, which we need to find," he informed her. As the technician kept the inverted eyelid in position with her thumb, the resident milked the conjunctiva down with two Q-tips, hand over hand, to expose the farthest superior recess of the conjunctiva. Joy felt the discomfort; more pus appeared. Then out came a hard half-inch-long object like a thin stick. When he rinsed it off, it was a broken piece of wood. He recognized it as part of a wooden Q-tip. "Look at this." He showed Joy and her mother the wood. "How in the world did this get there?"

THE EYE: WINDOW TO BODY AND SOUL

"Oh my god" was Joy's reply. "It's from one of my Q-tips. Sometimes I use a Q-tip to get a lost lens out of my eye."

The emergency room visit resulted in a rapid cure. Joy continued antibiotic drops two more days and was seen again in the MEEI residents' clinic. The supervising faculty, a middle-aged private practitioner from Boston, was pleased with the result—the patient was virtually cured—and amazed by the story. He praised the resident.

"You did a good job. There is no substitute for a thorough history and a very complete eye examination."

Chapter 3

THE TEACHER

Eye surgery is mostly taught by example. During the first year, a resident observes while assisting an experienced faculty surgeon, then during the next two years, a resident, always directly supervised by faculty, participates more and more, finally resulting in a scenario where the resident performs the operation and the faculty member assists. Then there is the gradation of difficulty. Not until residents have demonstrated ability to perform an easy case, such as the suturing of a facial laceration around the eyes, do they progress to other extraocular procedures, such as enucleation (eye removal) for cancer, cosmesis, or because the eye is already blind and painful. In such cases, vision is not at stake, and were there some error during surgery, it could easily be corrected. Finally, the resident begins to do intraocular operations, where a misstep, even a small one, can have disastrous and permanent consequences.

Of course, before residency, during the last year of medical school and the next very important year of surgical internship, students already get much experience in the surgical arena, often in the emergency room. Thus, by the time they enter ophthalmology, they already know sterile technique, suturing, and knot tying. However, the scale of their surgery is large, and now they have to adjust to a miniature environment where arm movements are eliminated, wrist movements minimized, and finger movements accentuated while peering through a microscope at a much-magnified view of a very small world.

There are statistics on the efficacy of this learning method. For example, the complication rate of cataract surgery done by residents is only slightly higher than that of their teachers. This difference disappears quickly and, by the third year of residency, has vanished. Because the surgical faculty, if properly chosen, often has a complication rate that is lower than that of nonteaching ophthalmic surgeons. The transient increase of serious complications by beginning residents is virtually negligible.

It is thus critically important that the teacher of eye surgery be a superb technician, who is thoroughly experienced and has the patience and nurturing ability to teach without making the student nervous and prone to error. John Peder, one of my own teachers, was such a surgeon. He was a short, stocky man of Polish origins, strong with broad shoulders, balding with a dapper moustache, and thick curly hair on his arms and chest, as you could tell when he wore his V-necked surgical shirt. Even in surgical cap and gown, his erect posture, with head held high, bespoke a formality of social mannerisms mirrored in the meticulous couture of his daily dress.

He was born as Johannes Pederovsky but had changed his name to simplify it. One of his professors had also recommended the change to avoid the Polish stereotyping of the early twentieth century in America, which the professor thought might interfere with building a successful medical practice. Dr. Peder had a resonant voice and always spoke slowly with every word deliberately chosen. His vocabulary was rich and his pronunciation precise, with just the right emphasis. It was a pleasure to hear him speak, and he was accustomed to the attention of his audience.

He was a wonderful demonstrator of surgical technique. His manipulation of fine ophthalmic instruments seemed intuitive, as if he had invented them. As his body remained still and only his hands, and occasionally his wrists, moved, every motion was as deliberate and controlled as the sonorous voice describing the movements in symphonic language. He liked having the same resident assigned to him twice weekly in the operating room for three months so that he could plan the gradual maturing of the surgical student precisely. He taught not only how to operate but also how to love the beauty of the surgical experience, the intricacies of instrument design, the interaction between different consistencies of the delicate, pliable tissues and hard metal. The proper use of curved scissors to make an incision into the peripheral cornea at the start of a cataract operation was a poetic experience.

During the 1960s, cataract surgery, the most common form of eye operation we had to learn, was very different from today. Removal of an opaque lens was done in toto—the entire lens as well as its capsule were taken out in one piece. Knowing that even if a small particle of the lens, pure protein, was left behind, we knew that a severe antigenic reaction might ensue, which could inflame the eye severely and risk the chance of a good visual outcome. Inflamed eyes are swollen, inside and out, and edema of the cornea as well as the retina are incompatible with good vision.

The lens, once removed, was not replaced so that strong spectacles or contact lenses were required to correct the vision postoperatively. Today, the operation has evolved into a totally different scenario, made possible by smaller sutures and needles, the use of ultrasonic fragmentation of the lens, and the development of intraocular lenses for insertion into the same space where the cataractous lens was located. However, even this operation continues to change with the development of evaporative lasers, which can remove the lens without utilizing the disruptive forces of ultrasound. With all this continual development, one aspect has not changed: the requirement for eye surgeons to be versatile and comfortable in the miniature world of fine manipulation and high magnification.

During the early 1960s, discussions of surgical technique for cataract usually involved the pros and cons of sliding versus tumbling the lens out of the eye. The goal was to remove only the lens and nothing more. The vitreous gel, filling most of the eye behind the lens and flimsily attached to it by a few fibrils, should not be violated.

"Don't lose vitreous" was *the word*. Thus, after a seventy-degree semicircular incision was made at the edge of the cornea, the surface of the lens, now easily accessible through a dilated pupil, could be grasped with a tiny suction cup or forceps and pulled forward past the pupil and then slid sideways out of the incision, like sliding a disc from a DVD player or out of its envelope. Depending on the strength of the fibrillar attachment to the vitreous, however, this maneuver risked pulling on the gel, which, on its posterior surface, was also variously attached to the retina. Undesirable traction could thus be transmitted to the retina and in turn cause retinal tears. These then might lead to retinal detachment, as fluid from the eye would find its way through the retinal holes and lift up the delicate retina. In those days, a small but significant percentage of cataract operations did result in retinal detachment, so any discussion about avoiding this complication was worthwhile.

Dr. Peder had given the subject much thought and, together with some colleagues from Boston and New York, devised a technique of tumbling them, which minimized traction on the vitreous and on the retina. As he would apply the suction device to the front capsule of the lens, he gently rotated it toward himself and toward the superior incision so that the inferior part of the lens rose up, breaking its vitreous attachments, while he oh so slightly pushed the superior part of the lens back toward the vitreous with the intent of neutralizing any traction on the gel. In the right hands, this delicate maneuver did indeed diminish late retinal complications, and for several years, it became the preferred method of cataract surgery for many ophthalmologists. The first time that he demonstrated this technique to me in the operating room, the performance was perfect. He spoke calmly as he controlled his fingers in slow, mellifluous movements. The lens came out as if it tumbled out by itself, the harmony between the surgeon and eye was astounding to observe. He stopped for a moment and blinked before placing the closing sutures. I looked at him from the side and thought that I could see a tear in his eye—the experience had been so gratifyingly beautiful.

"That's the way to do it," he said.

Chapter 4

LOOK AND YOU SHALL FIND

You would think that after college, four years of medical school, one year of internship, and another three years of ophthalmology residency training, one would finally quit this educational marathon and start practicing medicine. But no, not in my case and also not in the case of about 50 percent of eye residents, who continue the seemingly endless drudgery. They take a fellowship lasting from one to three additional years. Why? There are many disparate reasons for this choice. Often, it has to do with money—being more marketable at a time when group practice is the rule and those groups want to have super specialists in every subspecialty within ophthalmology as they compete with other groups. In my case, as was usually the case in an academic career, it had to do with wanting to narrow my field, become trained by the best subspecialist around, ultimately become as good as my teachers, and then, as my mentor had done, not only practice but also perform research in order to advance the field, gaining new information and then teaching it to my own students. I had learned and seen in my own teachers, from my father onward, that this was the three-legged milk stool I wished to sit on: specializing, teaching, and research. Thus, early narrow focus was the road to academic success. There was plenty of time later, after becoming a professor, to broaden one's view again. In fact, truly successful doctors, scientists, or academics in any field are often expected not to be focused or superspecialized later in their careers. Even Einstein was assumed to have valid opinions on almost everything, including politics.

However, once an academician has become successful, I think it is probably wise to resist the temptation to teach outside one's world. Stick to what you know if you want to continue to be correct.

The fellowship I took was in the study of retinal disease and especially the surgical treatment of retinal detachment. The Massachusetts Eye and Ear Infirmary in Boston was the best place at the time, and I was fortunate to be accepted there. Each fellow stayed eighteen to twenty-four months with new ones coming and graduates leaving every six months. There were six of us at one time, and our days consisted of examining patients with retinal conditions, usually retinal detachments, in order to get them ready for surgery the next day. Other days we spent in the operating room assisting the Retina Associates, our teachers in surgery. On on-duty weekends, we made rounds, which meant that we, by ourselves, went around the infirmary to visit each of the thirty or so hospitalized patients who were recovering from their surgery. Our job was to draw each operated retina, which meant making an accurate sketch of the retina with colored pencils in the chart. The patient was supine in the bed, and we, wearing a leadlamp (indirect ophthalmoscope), walked from side to side to see every aspect of the inner eye through the patient's dilated pupil. This was really what we were learning: the use of the indirect ophthalmoscope to see great detail in the back of the eye. Because the light source of the instrument was attached to a headband, it left both of our hands free, one to hold a glass focusing lens and the other to manipulate the patient's swollen eyelids to optimize our view. It would take us five to fifteen minutes for each patient, so these rounds could last from three to five hours depending on the complexity of each eye exam and the additional needs of each patient. It was exhausting but exciting, since most patients were recovering well.

During the week, on days when we were assigned to patient examination, which really meant retinal drawings, we hung around the fellows' room in the rear of the retina clinic, waiting to receive the phone call to tell us where and when we had to draw a patient. While we waited, we also supervised the eye residents, who were on their three-month rotation through the retina clinic, located next door. These residents, usually in their second or third year, were being first introduced to the retina. They did not know much and were very inexperienced with our instrumentation, but they were smart, motivated, and could be taught quickly. Part of their enthusiasm also stemmed from the atmosphere in the fellows' room, a pleasant place for camaraderie and common interests, where they could always get help from someone who had been in their shoes not long before without going to the professor. The fellow thus provided a nonintimidating source of information, where minor concerns could be voiced and "stupid" questions could be asked.

On one morning, four of us were having our coffee in the fellows' room when Bernie, one of the residents, came in followed by a simply dressed, pretty young girl with short dark hair held back by a headband, who was leaning forward over a wide stroller to check the contents as she wheeled it into the room. We looked up as Bernie, half turning his head back toward the girl, said, "I want you to meet my wife and our brand-new twins." We, of course, got up and walked toward them, a little surprised by this personal interruption in our professional environment but pleased by this opportunity to see this resident in a family role. Usually, we never had a chance to know any of the residents as more than students, divorced from life's other realities, incomplete people in an artificial learning environment.

Bernie introduced us to Molly, his wife, and told us that the twin boys were now a month old and everyone was doing fine. Apparently, the fact that they were twins had been a surprise, because in Costa Rica, where she was from, ultrasound examinations in the early 1960s were not routine. She had spent the last three months with her mother in San Jose, and then she and her mother came to Boston, two weeks before she was due to have the baby in the United States. The

THE EYE: WINDOW TO BODY AND SOUL

pregnancy had been uncomplicated, and the delivery at the Boston Lying-In Hospital was also pretty easy, even though there were twins. Each baby had been small at birth but not premature. "Just about five pounds each," exclaimed Molly proudly. Her wrinkle-free, uncomplicated face shone. She was very pretty.

The six of us now stood around having two conversations, mostly ignoring the sleeping children. None of the four of us fellows had any children, and only Glenn was even married. We learned that Bernie and Molly had met in Boston when she was a foreign exchange student at Boston University two years before. Subsequently, he went to visit her in Costa Rica, where they later got married. She was still a Costa Rican citizen, but when they moved into an apartment on Beacon Hill, a fourth-floor walk-up on Spruce Street, she had been able to get a job at a publishing company around the corner editing some Spanish translations. She was certainly fluent in English and barely had a foreign accent, except that she enunciated her words more precisely than most Americans.

Their pleasant conversations led to some jokes about Bernie taking paternity leave and also about the real reason why they had come to the retina clinic to show off the children, who had now woken up and were looking around at these noisy, laughing adults.

"You know, when you have a new child, you should always check on two things, the heart and the eyes. Make sure that there is no heart murmur and dilate the pupils—make sure that the retina is okay, especially with twins or prematures," Mort stated pompously.

"Isn't that why you came here, uh, to see us experts?"

Bernie paid little attention but Molly looked at him quizzically.

"Doesn't the pediatrician check all that?" she queried.

"Well, maybe the pediatrician can tell about the murmur, although they sometimes miss that as well, but they certainly can't see the retina, and they never dilate the pupil. But they wouldn't see it anyway, in all probability."

"What should we be looking for?" Molly wanted to know.

Now, Bernie spoke up, "I guess one thing is retinoblastoma, a tumor of young children, but it is very rare, but . . ." He hesitated. "It's probably a good idea to look . . . sometime."

"Listen," Mort spoke. "You're here now. It's very quick. We'll put this little eye drop—it doesn't sting—into both eyes, wait a few minutes, and then take a look. That's all there is to it."

"Are you sure it doesn't hurt?" Molly wanted to know.

"He's right," Bernie assured her. "We might as well just do it. Why not? We'll never get a better retina exam, and no, it doesn't hurt."

Glenn went to his desk to get the drops. "These are especially for children." Molly stepped back as Bernie held the lids open to let Glenn put one drop in each of the four eyes. The children remained quiet.

"You see, it doesn't even bother them."

We continued our conversations, with Molly staying close to the stroller and looking off and on at the undisturbed children. After a few minutes, Glenn checked to see if the pupils were getting larger.

"A few more minutes," he said.

When the pupils were about eight millimeters dilated, Bernie took the first of the children; swaddled him in a towel, which was used as a pillow cover on one of the exam tables; and let Glenn put in another eye drop of tetracaine in each eye to numb the eye surface. He then placed a small eyelid speculum, the size of a paperclip, between the lids to keep the eye open. He put his indirect ophthalmoscope on his head and adjusted it so the binocular view was perfect. Bernie, with one hand on the papoosed baby, was stroking his son's cheek with one finger of his other hand.

As Glenn looked in, he right away blinked his eyes a few times, as if his vision was blurry, then he looked again and turned to me.

"Would you mind taking a look? I am not sure what I am looking at." As he handed the scope to me, he looked at me directly, and I could see he was upset. Bernie, meanwhile, was busy stroking his child's cheek. When I looked, it was unmistakable, a pea-sized round white mass sticking up from the center of the retinal surface. Could

THE EYE: WINDOW TO BODY AND SOUL

this be a retinoblastoma? There was no other abnormality around it, no blood vessel distortions, no retinal detachment.

"Bernie, your child has something in his eye. Take a look."

By now, Molly, who had been away from the child, standing near the door, said, "What, what, what? What is it?"

"Let me take a look, Mol," He quickly took my scope and put it on his head. Being a resident who was still somewhat unaccustomed to the instrument, he was clearly slower in the adjustment of the light than he wanted to be. Impatiently, he took his first imperfect glance into the eye.

"Oh my god!" he exclaimed. "He has a tumor."

During the next half hour, both parents needed to be calmed down. Much reassurance was achieved by calling to have Dr. Charles Reagan, one of our mentors, come to the clinic. He was the one who always dealt with the retinoblastoma patients. He could tell us what this white lesion really was. Meanwhile, we did the job for which we were being trained. Glenn and I got out our clipboards and colored pencils, just as we would have for any patient before our professors came to check, and made accurate drawings of all four eyes of the children. Astoundingly, each of the four eyes had abnormal findings. Each eye had at least one white tumor and then some other smaller less-white-and-more-grey translucent bumps on or in the retina. Bernie stood by as we went about our business and then showed him what we were able to see.

When Charlie Reagan came, an hour or so later from the office around the corner, he immediately showed his mastery of the situation so that, within an hour, he was able to confirm our diagnosis of bilateral multifocal retinoblastoma in both children. His confident and calm manner bestowed some control over Bernie and Molly. He made a plan: x-rays (MRI did not exist), spinal taps, some blood studies, and a complete physical exam by a pediatric oncologist. The next day, he scheduled an examination under anesthesia of both children, which also permitted him to treat the tumors at the same time. As it turned out, because of the large size of the tumor in one eye of each child, those two eyes were enucleated (removed), and the few small tumors in the other eye of each child were treated with cryotherapy, a localized freezing technique. Because ball implants were used in the empty sockets, the cosmetic appearance of the children was excellent.

As we heard many years later, both boys grew up to be good students with no further problems until, twenty-six years later, one of them developed a bone cancer (osteosarcoma) of the upper leg, which was successfully treated and went into remission. Interestingly, now, fifty years later, one child has a successful career as a geneticist at the University of Texas in San Antonio, and the other became a pediatrician in Boston.

Since bilateral retinoblastoma is often genetically transmitted as a dominant trait, it was decided, after obtaining a negative family history from both Molly and Bernie, that they should both have thorough retina examinations themselves. Bernie was found to be normal, but Molly had a large white scar in the periphery of her right retina, not affecting her vision. She had never really had an eye exam before and had always had excellent vision. At first, she was surprised to hear about the scar, but later, as she told Bernie, she vaguely remembered that she had some eye problems as a small child. However, her parents had died when she was five years old during a revolution in El Salvador, after which her aunt and uncle in Costa Rica adopted her. When she contacted her uncle at the request of Dr. Reagan, he confirmed that when she was very little, her parents had taken her to a famous Boston-trained eye doctor in Guatemala, where she was treated. Now she remembered!

Later, Bernie asked Molly, "Why didn't you ever tell me about your eye problem?"

"I barely remembered," she said. "And I was fine and could see great. I thought it was unimportant, and I had almost forgotten about it." And then, she added, "Would you have married me if you had known?"

Chapter 5

THE LEARNING PROCESS

As first year residents, we were each assigned to a clinical faculty member, usually an ophthalmologist from the community who volunteered to teach in return for admitting privileges at the university hospital. Daily requests for consults from other departments were phoned in asking us to see patients who had developed eye problems. This day, Dr. Clarke, a third-year medical student, and I went to the bedside of an elderly lady, who had been in the surgical recovery room for thirty-six hours. At that time, in the early 1960s, intensive care units did not generally exist.

She was small and gray with disheveled hair and looked tiny in the messy large hospital bed. Her eyes were closed, and she moaned continuously. Her head sunk deep into the pillow while she fidgeted with the bed sheet, which she had pulled up under her chin as if she wanted to hide. Her swarthy complexion and the occasional "Mama" in her moans suggested that she was Italian—a good guess in the city of New Haven, where one-third of the population heralded from Southern Italy.

The surgical resident who had operated on this indigent patient for gallstones came over from another beside to explain that, following the laparoscopy to remove the gallbladder, the patient had never really woken up but continued to be stuporous. He had consulted neurology because he had noticed that her pupils were unequal and her right pupil, larger than the other one, was not reactive, not constricting, when he shone his penlight into the eye. He was sure that she had had a stroke. The neurologist had not yet seen the patient, and we, who had been asked to confirm the inequality of the pupils, were there first. This was not unusual: neurology and other nonsurgical specialties always took their time to do consults. Surgeons, possibly less contemplative and more action-oriented, usually showed up within twenty-four hours.

Indeed, the pupils were different sizes. I watched Dr. Clarke gently lift both upper lids with his thumb and forefinger as we all looked. The patient winced and let out a high-pitched whine. Yes, the right pupil did not move with light. His finger slipped, and the lid came down again. He repositioned his hand, and as he lifted the right lid again, the patient again acted as if in pain.

We tried to speak to the patient, but she seemed not to understand us. For the next few minutes, Dr. Clarke spoke about stroke and how it could affect pupillary responses. When he stopped his minilecture, he asked if we had questions. I wanted to know what nervous pathway was involved and whether he could tell where in the brain the stroke was. The young medical student wanted to know why the patient seemed to have pain when lifting the eyelid and also asked, "Why is the right eye red, or isn't it?"

"Take another look," Dr. Clarke told me. I lifted up one lid at a time and confirmed that the conjunctiva on the right side seemed redder than the left. There was also a different feel to the eye when you lifted the lid. Was the right eyeball harder than the left? I tested it several times as the poor patient moaned. Dr. Clarke watched me. He then felt the hardness of the eyes himself, pressing his forefinger to indent it, like feeling the pressure of a bicycle tire. "I think you are right. This patient has acute glaucoma with a mid-dilated and fixed pupil and may not have had a stroke after all!"

As it turned out, with the help of the patient's daughter's Italian translation, the diagnosis of acute angle closure glaucoma was confirmed in the eye clinic. Apparently, during the gallbladder surgery, the patient had been given atropine, a routine drug used in abdominal surgery to decrease bowel motility but which also dilated the pupils. In patients with small eyes and narrow angles, the slow recovery from this dilation can cause an acute rise in eye pressure, which makes the eye painful, red, and with a nonreactive mid-dilated pupil (unlike the more widely dilated pupil, which can accompany a stroke). In our scenario, a fragile old non-English-speaking patient was incorrectly labeled as stuporous, likely the result of stroke.

In this case, the simple, innocent question of an observant medical student saved the patient an uncomfortable, unnecessary, and expensive neurological workup and permitted us to treat her acute glaucoma in time to save her vision.

Chapter 6

CAN YOU SEE?

Suzan

She was in her late fifties, well beyond the age when the lens of the eye loses its elasticity and can no longer thicken to focus on nearby objects—a loss of accommodation for near, as we call it. She had always been a single woman, a tomboy, a marathon runner early on, a hiker, a swimmer, and lately a golfer. She had learned early to compete with her two brothers and usually beat them at most sports. She had entered a man's profession and became a dentist at a time when the only other women in dentistry were hygienists.

Although she never married—"Too busy," she said—she was not disinterested in men and did have boyfriends, some of whom lasted for years, but when interactions became too personal, she would suddenly end the relationship. Physically, she loved to be and do activities with people, but emotionally she was tough to get near. She loved winning a race and reaching the finish line but then disappeared into the crowd, avoiding social interaction. *She had nothing to fear,* I thought. She was athletic, good-looking, and professionally successful. She paid attention to her appearance and always wore clothes that complimented her athletic physique, her tan, her blue eyes, and her short curly salt-and-pepper hair. She never wore glasses.

Since she was a dentist, I had wondered about her vision without glasses at her age, when certainly she should have used some reading glasses or magnifiers for the close work she was performing on teeth. If she was nearsighted and wore a myopic prescription for distance vision, I could have understood it because then, simply taking her minus lenses off would have been equivalent to putting reading glasses (plus lenses) on so that she could focus on near objects. But she did not seem to have any regular distance glasses. Even her picture in the waiting room, hanging over her dental school diploma, showed no glasses, as did another photo of her crossing the finish line during a race. Could it be that she was nearsighted in one eye only, so she could see clearly at any distance with one eye at a time? I rejected that notion, since she obviously needed good binocular stereoscopic vision for her job.

Then one day, when I was the last patient, we walked out of the office together, and as she got behind the steering wheel, I saw her reach toward the dashboard and put on a pair of glasses. Amused, I knocked on her window. As she opened it, she took her glasses off again. "What is it?" she asked.

I answered, "You know, I'm an ophthalmologist, and I have always wondered why you didn't wear glasses. Do you mind, just to satisfy my curiosity, showing me those glasses there in your hand?"

She obliged—"Sure"—and handed them to me. "I'm supposed to wear these when I drive. It says so on my license." I quickly looked through the lenses, holding them at arm's length from my eyes. She had a nearsighted prescription of at least three diopters. This meant that without glasses, she could see perfectly at near. It also meant that without her prescription, everything beyond one-third of a meter, or about one foot away, would be blurry. Apparently, for whatever reason, she was willing, for most of her life, to live in a blur. If tested without her correction, she would have seen about 20/200 at far, good enough to qualify for legal blindness. Thank God that she at least wore her glasses while driving.

"Thank you," I said. "Sorry to be so nosy, but you have solved my little mystery. But don't you want to wear these glasses all the time? They make you see so much better, and they look good on you."

"No," she said, shaking her head. "I can see just fine without them."

Antonio

Olivia Pavane, a small woman of Mediterranean ancestry, came to the office with her twelve-year-old son Antonio. The child was well behaved, and when I greeted him, he said "Hello, sir"—a pleasant surprise when politeness seems to have become a lost art among children, especially teenagers, in the presence of adults. He had a slight build, was thin, with olive skin, had dark hair, dark eyes, and prominent eyebrows. No taller than his five-foot mother, he had not yet had his pubescent growth spurt. Yet his manner seemed mature, and he looked me directly in the eye when we spoke. His mother let him talk without interruption as he told me his history. The school nurse had sent him to an optometrist because he failed his eye exam, and the optometrist had been unable to get him to see better than 20/200, the big *E* on the Snellen chart.

"Are you a good student?" I asked.

He nodded and said, "Yes, sir," with emphasis on the *sir*.

"Where do you sit in the classroom?" I wanted to know.

"Well, I . . . I like to sit up front, where I can see the best."

"What are your favorite subjects?"

"Well, math. I like math . . . and science."

"But what is your most favorite thing in school?"

"Sports" was the immediate response.

Now, his mother interrupted, "He plays baseball and is on the team, the youngest boy on the team. He is very good. He is their star hitter. His dad and I go to all the games. He's amazing." She spoke with a slight Italian accent and put an *uh* or *ah* vowel sound behind most nouns. She certainly was proud of her son, who looked at her while she spoke. He was smiling.

The eye examination was mostly normal. However, I could not improve his vision to better than 20/100, and that was with coaxing. This meant that he would have to get as close as twenty feet from something he wanted to see when others could have seen it from as far away as a hundred feet. My cajoling and patience made no difference. Without any prescription, he saw 20/200 in each eye, and with a very weak, insignificant prescription, he could only be improved one line on the chart to the 20/100 level. Thus, he was legally blind, unable to see clearly without additional magnification.

The retinal exam was also normal when I first looked, but then, on close inspection of his dark-red macula, the center of the retina, I could see a very faint, mottled pigmentation deposit, as if fine pepper had been sprinkled there. Also, I noticed that my focus on the retinal detail was made more difficult by the continuous tiny jiggly motion of his eyes, nystagmus, which I had not noticed before. That prompted my eureka moment, leading me to the next test, the Ishihara color vision plates. When he failed that test, it meant that he really was color-blind as well. I now guessed that he had a congenital problem with his macula, a congenital form of macular degeneration, which could significantly impair his functions later in life, never being able to drive and never being able to read without magnifiers.

After considerable discussion with the boy and his mother, trying not to upset them overly by the realization that he might never see properly, we agreed to send him to Boston for special testing at the Massachusetts Eye and Ear Infirmary. This would be very important to differentiate several similar eye conditions, some of which were progressive and would lead to total blindness, while others were stationary. After a few weeks, the report from Boston was that Antonio had BCM, blue cone monochromatism, a stationary retinal cone deficiency only affecting central and color vision.

During the next twenty years, I continued to have Antonio as a patient. By then, I had acquired all the special test equipment in our own office so that periodic visits to Boston became unnecessary. He had continued to be a high school baseball star hitter, went to college in the city, where he did not need a car, and then found a job teaching math at the same college from which he graduated. He went to many baseball games.

As I thought about him over time, I continued to wonder how he could have been such a great ball hitter with such poor central vision. He would never be able to see the ball clearly. Over the years, Antonio and I had several opportunities to discuss this question. I explained to him the differences between central and peripheral vision. I showed him that when he held one hand directly in front of him, it was relatively easy to see. Doing this, he was using his central retina, the so-called macula, which had specialized receptors cells called cones, which were able to see better than the less sensitive rest of the retina, where other visual receivers, the rods, were located. To test rod function, he could hold his other hand to the side while continuing to look straight at his first hand. He would then see his second hand out of the corner of his eye, but not as clearly. Those were his rods seeing the second hand. It was difficult at first to get him to understand this, because his cones were abnormal, and the difference between his side vision and his central vision was not as great as in normal patients, but he finally understood. What I could never make him comprehend was the difference between the color vision of cones and black-and-white vision of rods, because he had never seen true colors, just shades of blue.

"So where do you look," I asked him, "when someone pitches the ball and you are supposed to hit it?"

"I just look at the pitcher, and I guess I don't move my eyes very much" was the answer. "I can see the ball coming all the way. I don't have a problem." The latter was obvious. It reminded me of other patients, usually elderly people with macular degeneration—who have very poor central vision—who could not drive or read yet could detect a fly or ant walking across the carpet. When they then tried to look directly at it, they would not see it. These patients also had normal rods, normal peripheral vision, normal vision out of the corner of their eyes. Perhaps it was the bug's motion or the baseball's movement, as its image travelled across the peripheral retina, that made the patient see. Whatever the explanation, it gave me an additional appreciation for the complexity of blindness and how it affects different people so differently. Some of that difference is, of course, related to whether the blindness is congenital or acquired. It is difficult to miss something that you have never had.

Alexandra

She was formidable in her manner, unhesitating in her stride, and wore a business suit with a white shirt and tie. She was accompanied by a girl in her twenties carrying a bassinet. The girl's loafers, socks, plaid skirt, and white blouse looked like a uniform. When they sat down, a nippled bottle appeared in the girl's hand and was then plunged into the bassinet. Judging from the movement of the white blanket and some gurgling noises, the recipient of the bottle's contents was a baby. The woman paid little attention to the feeding and arose to find a magazine on the table. She then sat down, crossed her legs, and leafed through *Vanity Fair*, looking at the pictures. Her shoes had three-inch heels. Her comfort did not last long, as she was asked by the desk clerk, who peered down at her across the counter, to fill out some papers: disclaimers, a patient's bill of rights, a permission to share information, documentation of insurance, and a medical history—eight pages in all. As she sat down again, she held the clipboard at reading distance but then put it on her lap to distance herself from it as she leaned back. She used the attached pen to write but twice had to ask her au pair to read something for her because "this print is impossible to see. Why don't they make it legible?" The girl obliged.

The information she provided included that she was forty-four and married. She was the vice president of New England Bank Associates, a regional bank which had recently been in the news, having purchased the local Oliver Bank. She was apparently healthy and took few medications—Valium, periodically; Ambien for sleep;

aspirin; and multivitamins. Recently, she had stopped taking the pill, because she was too old to have children. She drank two glasses of red wine daily.

When the technician later questioned her, the Valium was only to calm her before a major speech, and the aspirin was "to be safe." Because she had left her au pair and her baby in the waiting room, she was agreeable with sharing other information. She spent the first twenty years of her career traveling the Western world for the Bank of America and then only recently settled down in Stamford, Connecticut, to get married. She had met this wonderful man, seven years younger, who was a playwright and stage director in New York. To her surprise, she got pregnant and had this late child, "which I certainly did not plan on. A little inconvenient—thank God I can afford help. Most of my married friends are grandmothers by now."

Recently, she had developed some vision problems with reading. "Things up close get blurry, but not all the time. Sometimes it's like seeing double, but not really. It makes me dizzy and feel funny, maybe nauseous, but then it goes away. I thought I should have it checked out. And my mother had some eye problems when she got older—glaucoma, cataract, or something. She was always fiddling around with several pairs of glasses, although she never had worn glasses before. She had glasses for reading, different ones for television, and another pair for playing bridge. She had glasses everywhere."

After the technician was finished with the history and the preliminary testing, she steered the patient into my room, where I was waiting. The chart indicated 20/20 distance vision, normal eye pressures, and no other perceived abnormalities. I looked at the patient and asked, "Are you here for your regular checkup, or do you have a particular problem?"

"Well, doctor, I have this new child, and when I hold it on my arm and look down at it, I feel sick to my stomach."

Joe

Joe Novack, a retired navy captain, with the blue eyes of a sailor peering from his tanned, leathery face, was finally paying more attention to himself. The crow's feet at his temples spoke of years of squinting at the horizon, and his US navy cap, from which he was inseparable, testified to his love of navy life and of the sea. He could tell navy stories forever.

He had recently lost his wife to ovarian cancer. The last years had been tough, with radiation, chemotherapy, constant worry, and doing most of the housework, including the cooking. Finally, hospice took over—almost against his will—when pain, incontinence, and bedsores required more care than he could deliver.

Although his navy career had included many periods, months at a time, when he was not with his wife, he now suddenly felt lonely for female companionship. At hospice, he had met a beautiful blond woman, Barbara, whose much older husband was also a hospice patient. At first, Joe had thought that she was visiting her father, but no, this was her second husband, whom she had married in her late thirties after her first husband had died in a skiing accident. At that time, her only child, a daughter, was eighteen and a freshman in college. The shock of the accident and the financial burden of college tuition both conspired to discover a savior—a newly retiring sixty-one-year-old widower who had been a vice president at the local bank, whose advice she had sought to manage her finances. The rescue was mutual, and the next twenty years were comfortable and calm for both. Now, at eighty-one, he was dying, having had several small strokes—the consequences of which were difficult to differentiate from the symptoms of his Alzheimer's disease.

Both Joe's wife and Barbara's husband died the same week. Being busy with all the related arrangements, they went their own ways and did not encounter each other for two months. Then, Joe telephoned Barbara, getting her phone number from hospice, which was, at first, reluctant to give out this information. He had to convince the hospice office manager that this had nothing to do with patient confidentiality.

He and Barbara were not patients, and he fibbed he had something of Barbara's that he needed to return to her, something personal.

Barbara seemed glad to hear from him, and they agreed to have lunch. Six months later, they were married. He, now seventy-four, was delighted with the prospect of sharing the last years of his life with this beautiful younger, seemingly uncomplicated woman, whose affectionate manner and carefree spirit elevated his mood to a level he had not experienced for years. She also felt liberated and comforted by his apparent devotion to her. They did everything together and seemed inseparable, like young lovers. One highlight of their day was to sit on a small dune, just above the beach, from five till seven o'clock at sunset, with him peering from under his navy cap at the horizon, pointing out an occasional passing ship, and telling stories of the sea. Meanwhile, she listened as she managed the provisions—vodka tonics, crackers, and cheese—and used the top of the cooler as a table.

It was during this period in their lives that he, for the first time in years, permitted himself the luxury of self-reflection. He now realized that his vision had been bothering him and not just recently. At first, it was just during night driving, when the light of oncoming cars seemed too bright, harsh, and dazzling. Later, the glare became blinding, and he avoided driving after dusk. He now also noticed an uncomfortable silver sheen over everything, especially on sunny days. When the sky was gray but bright, colors were hard to see. An optometrist, years before, had warned him about early lens changes, so he now thought that he was developing cataracts. His suspicions were confirmed by an ophthalmologist, and soon thereafter, he was scheduled for cataract surgery, the right eye first and then the left eye one week later. His preoperative vision was 20/50, four lines worse than the 20/20 line of the Snellen eye chart. It was definitely time to get this problem fixed.

The first operation was so easy for him that he could hardly believe it. Barbara took him to the surgicenter. He signed some documents, got partially undressed, and sat on a large stretcher chair. They covered him with a blanket. An IV was started, and he joked with the nurse who had also taken his blood pressure. That was the last thing he remembered until he heard Barbara's voice. She was getting instructions about the eye patch, the protective plastic eye shield for bedtime use, and the installation of some eye drops. They were home a little after noon. During the next six days, until the left eye would be operated, he noticed the gradual improvement of his vision, which was now clearly better than his left eye. Most of the time, however, he kept the shield taped across his eye, which was more comfortable and also alleviated the concern that he might rub it during one of his daily naps. Barbara enjoyed playing the nurse role, and he acquiesced to being a ready patient.

The second operation was even less stressful, now that he was familiar with the routine. He felt so good when they returned home in the middle of the day that they went to the beach at five o'clock to reclaim their cocktail-hour habit, which they had not done for a week. The protective plastic shield, which had small holes in it through which he could see, was over his right eye, and a patch was over the left.

The next day, after brushing his teeth and removing his eye shield and patch, he looked around and out the window. The bright low sun did not bother him like before. Everything was so bright and clear, so blue and without uncomfortable glare. He felt reborn, not believing the improvement in his vision. He could even see more dirt on the windowpanes. He leaned forward to look at himself in the mirror. "Barbara, honey, come here!" he shouted into the bedroom.

"What is it, baby?" she said as she quickly came in.

"My face," he said, palpating his cheek with two fingers. "I've got all these black lines—so many of them. What did they do to me?"

"Nothing, baby, you're fine. It's just one or two wrinkles. Why don't you look at me?" He turned to look. "Well actually, you don't look so good either."

W. A. J. VAN HEUVEN, M.D.

Veronica

An obese mother, appearing to be in her forties, with disheveled shoulder-length streaked blond hair, wearing a sweatshirt, short shorts, and flip-flops, came with her daughter, our patient. Veronica, eleven years old according to the patient list, was thin but healthy-looking, with short dark hair, and tidily dressed in a white T-shirt, shorts, and sneakers. She seemed undisturbed by the loud talking and laughing of her mother on her cell phone. Another patient in the waiting room, a middle-aged man reading a book, looked up, grimaced, got up, walked to the end of the short hallway leading to the offices, and began studying the series of diplomas and membership documents of the practicing doctors, displayed to attest to their training, expertise, and experience. One of the technicians, observing the discordant scenario through the receptionist's window, went to the waiting room to retrieve the two women and put them in a newly vacated exam room.

"Ma'am, please turn off your cell phone. We are now going into the doctor's office."

The mother quickly terminated her conversation. "I'll call you back when we're finished here."

As she placed her phone into the oversized pocketbook, she pulled out a magazine in the same movement and, as soon as she slumped into the corner chair, began flipping noisily through its pages, not looking at any page long enough to get more than a glimpse of the pictures of scantily dressed unnaturally thin women.

Veronica sat down carefully on the exam chair, facing me, looking up in anticipation.

"Well, what's the matter? What brings you here?" I asked.

"I see blurry, and I have headaches."

Now the mother interrupted, "She's been having headaches for a while now, at least a year."

"Was there anything going on in her life that could have started the headaches? Was she sick? Did she have a cold? And where are the headaches? Can you point to them?"

Veronica raised both arms and pointed to her temples.

"And then, also here in the back of my head," she said as she touched the upper part of her neck. She was speaking softly.

The eye examination that ensued was entirely normal, except that her vision was 20/70 in each eye. Suspecting nearsightedness, I performed a quick refraction but still could not improve her vision, no matter how hard I tried. She was not myopic. Finally, I even resorted to a combination of plus and minus lenses, totaling zero power to try to uncover willful malingering. She was not fooled. Her vision remained 20/70. Rechecking, her pupils reacted normally and equally to light. Then, I decided to test her color vision using multicolored charts (Ishihara plates) showing numbers in one set of colors against a background of other colors.

Initially, she could not identify any numbers. Then, with some kind encouragement and a little patience by me, she performed increasingly better and finally got them all. Before dilating her pupils, I ordered a visual field test to see if any particular part of her visual pathway from the eyes to the brain was abnormal. For example, some children can develop an optic nerve problem, but this tends to occur only in boys and is hereditary. There was no history of such a condition, the mother confirmed, as the girl was taken to another room by the technician. While she was being tested, the mother and I had the opportunity to discuss additional history of potential importance.

"Did Veronica eat normally?"

"Absolutely, she eats as much as I do, and look at me" was the answer.

"Did she ever smoke, or did you ever suspect her to be taking any drugs? Was there marijuana in the house or anything else addictive? Did she have any close friends who might be taking illegal drugs?"

The answers were a resounding no to all the questions.

"What was the family situation like? Was Veronica happy?"

"We are all happier now," the mother volunteered. "Two years ago my husband—he was a forester—died in a motorcycle accident. It was a terrible shock. Veronica was very close to him. He would take her on weekends to tromp through the woods as he marked trees for cutting. She really learned a lot about trees and nature and things. In winter, they'd do it on snowshoes. I never had to worry about her when she was out with her dad."

"I'm sorry to hear that. So how is she now?"

"Well, she's okay . . . I guess she's better. After the accident, we couldn't afford to keep up the house, an old farmhouse. We sold it pretty quickly and moved in with my sister, who also has a child about the same age, actually a little older. She is a single mom, so we've got four women in one house. I thought that it would be good for Veronica to have someone near her own age to talk to, other than just me. The two girls share a bedroom, but it hasn't always worked out. With all this puberty stuff going on in my niece, they don't seem to have too much to talk about."

When Veronica came back to the exam room, I saw that the visual field test was normal. There was no sign of decreased sensitivity in her central vision and no sign of the hereditary optic neuropathy, toxicity of any kind, or nutritional vitamin deficiency, all of which might produce uncorrectable vision loss. The dilated retina and optic nerve exam, which I did next, also showed nothing abnormal.

"You did a great job on that test," I told Veronica. "You must be smart. Aren't you pretty good in school?"

She nodded yes.

"I think you are going to be just fine. This happens sometimes, but it goes away. But we do want to take a little blood and some urine too, just to be sure. Do you mind?"

The technician took Veronica to another room so that I had a further opportunity to talk to the mother.

"The tests are just to make sure that I'm not missing anything. I think they'll be normal. There is really nothing wrong with her eyes. It may just be stress. She can't help it. She just lost her father, then her home, and then even you, her mother, in a way. At least she's lost your full attention, now that you are living with other people, even if they are family. They say that moving or losing your home is one of the most stressful things that can happen to a person. Well, Veronica has lost a lot more than just her home. What she needs now is lots of

THE EYE: WINDOW TO BODY AND SOUL

love, lots of hugs, lots of special attention from you and maybe from your sister too. Talk to her about it, if you have a chance. It's not likely that Veronica will get much of what she needs from your niece. That girl has her own problems, going through puberty!"

When Veronica came back with the tech, we told her we would see her again in ten days, after the tests results were available. I told her that her eyes were fine and that her blurry vision would clear up.

"Think of it as having a cold in your eyes. Colds are temporary. There is no treatment for them, but they clear up. Just give it a little time, and good luck in school. You're smart, I know, so you're probably at the top of your class. Your vision is going to be just fine to keep that up, I promise!"

When the mother and daughter returned ten days later, Veronica's vision had improved slightly to 20/40, the same in both eyes. However, testing her acuity at near, using a reading card with small print, she could see 20/20. The eye exam was again normal. The blood tests for vitamin B levels were normal, as was the urine test for toxic substances. Her headaches were still bothering her some, but not as often. To my surprise, at her mother's urging, she had started to show up for field hockey practice after school. Quite often, her mother would come to watch before practice was finished, since she had to come to school anyway to pick up her daughter, who by then had missed the regular school bus.

Six weeks later, Veronica's vision had improved to 20/20. She had also become more talkative. She was excited because, after their office visit with me, they were going shopping to decorate her new room. Apparently, her mother had vacated a small room next to her own bedroom, which she had used as a closet.

"I'm going to make it just beautiful," she said, smiling at me really for the first time.

I saw them twice more during the next few months. Veronica's vision remained stable at 20/20, and her headaches slowly dwindled. Neurological testing and an MRI of the brain, which would have been the next step if the symptoms had not cleared, were not needed. The mother's cell phone was never heard again in our office.

Chapter 7

A New Disease

In 1981, when I was an associate professor teaching eye residents, I frequently crossed paths with the chief resident of the Internal Medicine Department, whom I thought to be slated for an academic career himself. Not only was he very well-informed and obviously smart, but he also had an exceptionally good bedside manner and effused genuinely kind and compassionate behavior toward patients and their families. He already was a wonderful teacher of other residents, which included our ophthalmic residents, because internal medicine and ophthalmology had so many patients in common.

During that year, I got to know Jeff Ferguson pretty well since our schedules seemed to be similar: morning rounds on the same ward between 7:00 and 8:00 AM and lunch in the doctor's cafeteria around 12:30 PM. He was raised in Southern California, where his father was a family practitioner in Ventura, not far from Los Angeles. He had come East for his college education at Yale and then returned to UCLA for medical school at his father's request, but then he returned to the East for his internship in New York City and a residency at Albany Medical College, within easy reach of the big city, which he loved because of the theater, the opera, and especially the ballet.

Once, when he joined me at an empty seat at a small lunch table, he asked politely, "Do you mind if I join you?" a boyish smile on his rosy-complected face. He told me that he had first wanted to become a ballet dancer after seeing Rudolf Nureyev perform in Los Angeles. He was twelve at the time and was instantly mesmerized by the powerful yet graceful leaps and turns of the dancer. Somehow, he knew he could do that too. He convinced his mother to send him to ballet school, but it didn't last long. The trip from Ventura to Los Angeles twice a week became too burdensome for the family, he was ridiculed by some of his male classmates, and his father became increasingly skeptical about this activity for his only son, whom he thought should get more serious and aim for a professional career, hopefully in medicine.

"So how did you end up in Albany?" I asked. "Why not New York City? There are at least a dozen residencies in the city that you could have taken."

"Yes, I know, but I am close enough to the city so I can go there whenever I want whenever I have a weekend off. And then I have a great friend who is doing a dermatology residency here. He also loves the performing arts, especially Broadway theater. We try to arrange our schedules so we have the same weekends off so we can go to New York together. We take the early Saturday morning train, check into the Taft Hotel, just a few blocks from Times Square and the theater district, and we're off! We usually see two plays and one ballet before coming back on the Sunday evening train, after the matinee. It works out great and—" he paused while pulling a weekly *Variety* from his white-coat pocket—"this is what keeps me going the rest of the time." He smiled, and a blush came over his young face, which made him look like a little boy.

"Well, aren't you lucky to have such a good friend and companion?"

As the weeks passed, I continued to bump into Jeff and was able to compliment him on his teaching of our eye residents, especially in the emergency room, which was the source of many eye consults to and from the Internal Medicine Department. Every time I saw him, I could see the top of the weekly *Variety* poking out of his white-coat pocket. I guess it kept him constantly up-to-date on the latest New

York entertainment news, theater reviews, box office results, and Broadway cover stories.

Then, one day, he called me because he had some eye symptoms that he could not explain.

"I am sorry to bother you, but I just wanted to know what is going on with my eyes. I can see just fine. You know that I don't wear glasses, but . . . I seem to get these flashes in my side vision, like someone has lit a sparkler. I don't see it all the time, but it seems to be there especially in the early morning and in the evening. It doesn't really bother me except that I never had this before."

"Do you ever have migraine headaches?" I asked.

"No, not really. In fact, I never have a headache at all."

"Do you think I could look at your eyes some time?" "Sure."

"Let's do that some time at the end of a day, when you do not have to work that night. I might have to dilate your pupils, which would blur your vision for a few hours."

The next afternoon at five thirty, just after medicine rounds, he showed up at my office. The eye exam went smoothly. His vision was excellent, and the external and pupil exams were normal, as were the eye pressures. A few minutes after instilling dilating drops, the pupils were large enough to observe much of the retina and optic nerve. At first glance, everything looked normal, but then, on closer inspection, there were two or three small white spots in each retina, which had the appearance of so-called soft exudates—tiny areas of retinal swelling, not specific for any particular disease but fairly common in a variety of conditions, many of which would never occur in such a young person. It prompted me to ask more questions about his medical history.

"Have you been sick recently?"

"Just a little. Three weeks ago, I had a cough which would not quit. My attending thought it might be pneumonia. He took an x-ray and gave me some erythromycin. Then it got better."

"You don't have diabetes, do you, or high blood pressure?"

"No to both."

"How about lupus?"

"I don't think so. I have no other symptoms or signs of it."
"Have you ever been tested for it?"
"No."
"How about Lyme disease? Have you been to any areas where it is endemic, such as Cape Cod, Nantucket, Martha's Vineyard, the New England coast, or even the town of Lyme itself?"
"No, I don't particularly like the coast, the salt water, or the beach. I burn too fast. My skin is too sensitive."
"I have one more question. I'm almost embarrassed to ask it because I know the answer already. Have you ever taken intravenous drugs—recreational drugs? You know what I mean."
"Absolutely not" was the quick response.
"Well then, let's do some blood work. I'll order a complete blood count to rule out anemia and other such things, a lupus test, a Lyme test, and a blood sugar. Then, we'll go from there, okay?"
"Sure."

Two days later, I had all the results. They were all normal or negative. It was a puzzle, so I decided to repeat the eye exam. This time, I pulled back the eyelids farther than before, while Jeff looked maximally in all directions to expose the conjunctiva as much as possible while I looked through the slit-lamp microscope. The only probably insignificant finding was a very small—less than one millimeter in diameter—red spot under his left lower lid, which I interpreted as a small vascular anomaly and nothing special.

I then dilated his pupils, but this time waited a full twenty minutes to permit maximal dilation, which gave me a much larger view of the retina than before. I paid special attention to the peripheral retina, which I had not examined previously. The right eye looked entirely normal, but to my surprise, the left peripheral retina showed two patches of white, each with irregular borders, and some flame-shaped hemorrhages on their edges. This was clearly an active process and very abnormal. Was this some sort of infection? I told Jeff of my finding and suggested that this retinal brushfire, as I named it, might easily explain his symptoms. Clearly, as it progressed, it would stimulate his retina, which would respond like any retina when stimulated, by sending a message to the brain, which would interpret it as light, just like all the other messages from the retina. What I did not know was what was causing the problem.

During the following hour, Jeff and I went over his history again to pinpoint a possible infectious cause. Had he traveled recently? Had he been to the San Joaquin Valley in California, where coccidiomycosis was endemic? What else could cause this? We came up with no answers.

It was clearly time to consult with his boss in the Internal Medicine Department. Jeff agreed and started to tell me all the different blood tests that should be ordered. I called Jeff's chairman, who was not immediately convinced of the importance of a massive diagnostic workup, but when I showed him photos of the retina and visual field—proof that some areas of the peripheral retina were no longer functioning—he became convinced of the urgency of the situation. During the next week, as blood tests were being done and a chest x-ray showed some pneumonia-like lung opacities, the retinal inflammation progressed slightly and new hemorrhages appeared. The small red vascular anomaly on the conjunctiva also became more prominent.

As it turned out, this was my first case of cytomegalovirus infection of the retina in an HIV positive patient with AIDS (acute immune deficiency syndrome). The conjunctival red lesion, which I had biopsied, was Kaposi sarcoma, and the lung changes were typical of pneumocystis pneumonia. In retrospect, it all fit: AIDS in a homosexual male patient who acquired it probably through sexual contact with his partner.

However, in 1981, this disease was just beginning to be described and had not even been officially named. In addition, it was not yet widespread, especially in our area of the country, where, as the only retina specialist around, I had never seen it. But that was barely an excuse for me not to make the right diagnosis. I had certainly heard about immune deficiency and retinitis, but in this case, it occurred in a colleague and friend, whose social history, although known to me, never even rang a bell in my brain that sexual transmission between males was involved. To me, the possibility that my friend was homosexual had never even entered my mind.

The story of Jeff Ferguson did not end well. He was treated with numerous drugs, some of them antiviral agents, and his retinitis resolved, his conjunctival sarcoma (cancer) did not recur, and his pneumonitis cleared up. Realizing the potential risk to his friend and partner, I made sure that he also was treated. A few months later, Jeff started to cough again and became hoarse. He was diagnosed with throat cancer and referred to Sloan-Kettering Hospital in New York City, where he was treated, both as an inpatient and as an outpatient, for the next year and a half, after which he died of metastatic cancer of the brain. He never did finish his last year of residency.

Those were the early days of AIDS, before any effective treatments were available.

Part II

Too Much Focus

Chapter 1: The Second Eye 49
Chapter 2: Routines 54
Chapter 3: Is this Research or What? 59

Chapter 1

THE SECOND EYE

The referral came from another retina specialist in a neighboring town some seventy miles away, because the patient wanted to be able to stay with her daughter, who lived in our city, following the surgery. This type of patient was also easy to refer because her retinal detachment was not one that any surgeon would want to tackle, a massively scarred, tightly puckered total detachment (so called PVR—proliferative vitreoretinopathy) which had developed after she fell on the front steps of her house. She had come down hard face first on the decorative brass knob at the end of the railing. Although the knob was designed to fit comfortably in the palm of the hand to facilitate a firm grasp, it was also the perfect size to fit the orbit between brow and cheekbone. Thus, as she fell, the impact to her eye was unchecked by the boney surround and resulted in a ruptured eyeball. She also broke her hip at the same time. The resultant repairs, which took several hours of operating time, had required considerable coordination between anesthesia, ophthalmology, and orthopedics so that her "open globe" could be repaired and her hip pins placed at the same time without the need of two separate anesthetic inductions.

It was now six weeks later. Mary was still in her wheelchair. She told me the story of her accident and how much it had hurt. The doctors had been wonderful, and she was out of the hospital in no time—two days. Her daughter had immediately come to fetch her and bring her to San Antonio, where she had been for the last six weeks, with an occasional car trip to her doctors for postoperative visits. Her hip was doing fine, but she still could not see out of her left eye. She had had previous cataract surgery in both eyes, which had resulted in excellent vision for driving "even without glasses, for the first time in my life!" she exclaimed. She did need reading glasses, however, and had several of them lying around the house. Then, she had special readers for her favorite pastime, crocheting, and another pair for playing bridge with her Wednesday group. Since the cataract operations, she had experienced seeing some "floaters once in a while, especially one large one off to the side." She moved her right hand to indicate the location. "But then, other times it's just a bunch of small black dots."

"How many?" I asked.

"Oh, I don't know. At least twenty."

"Do you know which eye they were in?"

"No, not really. They just float by, just like the big black one, my big black crow. They just fly by in one direction and then come back going in the other direction. Do you think it could be in my head?"

With difficulty, and causing some discomfort, we transferred Mary to an exam chair, which could be reclined so that a complete retina examination, using the head-worn indirect ophthalmoscope, could be performed. At this moment, it was important to shorten the exam as much as possible, because the patient was clearly experiencing hip pain, lying flat with her legs extended. Since she was only at my office for the specific purpose of scheduling an operation on her left eye, there was no real reason to prolong the patient's agony. However, possibly because a resident was with me, I did not permit myself to set a poor example and proceeded to be as thorough as I would have been without the extenuating circumstances of Mary's painful hip.

During the exam, I distracted her by obtaining some additional medical history about her family. Her father also had some retina problems in his late sixties. She didn't know what it was, but he lost his vision in one eye. He had also been very nearsighted, just as she was until her cataract surgery had corrected it. She remembered, as a little girl, sitting on her father's lap, playing with his glasses. Looking through them, she remembered that everything looked smaller.

The recollections seemed to pleasure her, and she temporarily forgot about her hip. It gave me the chance to repeat the same sentence that I always use with patients who had a serious monocular problem: "I know, Mary, that you are here for your left eye, but right now, your right eye is all you have, so in a way, your right eye is more important than your left. Therefore, I am now going to look at your right eye first, just to make absolutely sure that it is in great shape and that you will always have good vision at least in that eye." She agreed, realizing that she had no choice.

Thanks to her cooperation, with minimal squirming to keep her hip comfortable, the retina exam of the good eye took less than five minutes. In the far peripheral part of the retina, I found a large horseshoe-shaped retinal tear. Immediately, I recalled Mary's mention of the many spots she had seen in the past. It all fit perfectly with the diagnosis of vitreous detachment causing a retinal tear, which, in turn, could any day cause a retinal detachment in that normal eye as well.

I explained to Mary the whole sequence of events that had happened in her eye. "The vitreous gel fills up most of the eyeball. In the back of the eye, it lies up against the retina, which is the layer which with you see, like the film in a camera, where images are focused. Well, the vitreous gel, during a lifetime, starts to liquefy from the inside out. By the time a person is sixty-five or so, it will become a liquid-filled balloon, with only the skin of the balloon being made of rubbery gel. At some point, that skin gets so thin that it breaks, and the balloon collapses, all within the eye. At that moment, the sticky surface of that balloon suddenly pulls away from the retina. In most patients, this happens without causing a problem. The only thing that patients notice is perhaps some flashes of light and a few floaters. The light flashes are due to the transient traction on the retina as the vitreous surface pulls away. The floaters are a few pieces of material, some small cells or fibers, which are sheared off the retina. In some patients, and this apparently happened in your right eye, the vitreous collapse—we call it a vitreous detachment—caused a complication. As it happened, there must have been an unusually strong adhesion between the vitreous surface and the retina in one small area, so when the vitreous detached, it tore the retina. You now have a situation where you have a hole in the retina and watery gel next to that hole. This is the perfect setup for a retinal detachment. The liquid starts to go through the hole and lifts up the retina, separating it from the next layer under the retina where most of the retinal blood vessels are. Without those blood vessels providing nutrition, your retina dies, and the eye becomes blind."

Mary listened intently to my explanation, which was also meant to be heard by the resident. Then, I looked once more at all 360 degrees of the peripheral retina to be certain that no other tears existed. She seemed gratified by the thoroughness of the exam and would have tolerated even more discomfort if it had been necessary. She was not upset when I told her that this retinal tear was now a priority and needed to be fixed right away, even before we tackled the other eye. It was simply too dangerous to wait. I could seal the tear with a laser right away in the office. Even though it is never a good idea to give any patient a guarantee of success, I assured her that the laser would prevent a retinal detachment in her good eye. The laser treatment was done uneventfully, and Mary expressed her delight that I had found something that could be fixed.

The following day, we operated on the injured eye, a long and difficult procedure, with limited immediate success: a partial reattachment of the retina. A few weeks later, however, the retina redetached again totally. At the time, the retina was so severely scarred and puckered that I considered it inoperable. For a while, she had light perception vision only. Then, she became totally blind in that eye.

Now, five years later, I still see her periodically to check on her good eye. Every time, she reminds me of that first day, "Dr. van Heuven, I am so glad that you looked at my other eye."

"Me too," I agreed, continuing to wonder why the referring retina specialist had never mentioned the large tear in her good eye. Had he never looked at that good eye? Had he been only focused on the obvious problem?

Chapter 2

Routines

The system in the office was rigorous. It optimized efficiency, as was immediately apparent in the brusque, almost humorous no-nonsense manner of Miss O'Brien, the Irish nurse who was the first staff to interact with every patient. It accommodated a large number of referrals without sacrificing excellence for speed. The system protected the doctors so that they were never rushed and could pay all their needed meticulous attention to detail. People with retinal detachment were sent to the Retina Associates from all over the world to benefit from the latest and best surgical expertise anywhere. When they came, they found a group of four highly focused physician-surgeons using newly improved diagnostic methods and recently invented surgical techniques. They also found that this was the training ground for the world's future retina surgeons who, once graduated from the fellowship, would fan out worldwide to spread the gospel.

I was one of six fellows to spend $1-1/2$ years in this environment. One of us would arrive every three months when another would graduate, so there were always different levels of experience among the fellows. We had a thoroughly prescribed schedule. Some days, we saw mostly new patients, and other times we were assigned to the operating room. Every effort was made to let us assist in the surgery

THE EYE: WINDOW TO BODY AND SOUL

of the same patient we had worked up earlier. I particularly remember Mr. Alan Peszinski, a retired accountant from New York, who was a morning patient seen by one of the Associates and who needed to be readied for surgery the next day. Miss O'Brien had already taken a brief medical history and performed the initial basic testing. His vision was light perception only with a faint hint of seeing some hand movements in the eye with the retinal detachment, but an excellent 20/20 in the other eye. My mentor had confirmed the diagnosis, and now it was up to me to complete the history and the physical examination, the most important part of which was doing a retinal drawing.

Mr. Peszinski had been an accountant for forty-six years, ever since graduating from college. Numbers were his game, and he was able to do much of his work from home, since he needed no coworkers, doing the accounting for a six-store chain of small Brooklyn grocery stores all by himself. Most of the work was handwritten, but once a year he would get out the typewriter to fill out the tax forms. His days were repetitive and predictable. While his wife did the housework, he mostly sat at his desk by the window, from which he could see the corner of the city park diagonally across the street. Four times a day, he walked his dog Max to that park, chatted briefly with some other dog walkers whom he had met over the years, and went back to his desk. After his lunch sandwich, which he shared with his wife, he took a twenty-minute nap and then resumed creating the large spreadsheets of daily expenses and income for each of the six stores. Evenings were spent watching television.

The Peszinskis had one daughter, who was now in her thirties and married. Her son Mackie was five years old and had recently been given a toy kaleidoscope for his birthday. He brought it with him to show his grandfather at the traditional Sunday family lunch. Mackie was mesmerized by the ever-changing color pattern as he turned the tube while looking through the small hole at the end. When Alan looked with his left eye at first, he couldn't see anything, so he switched to the right eye and immediately saw the changing symmetrical display. He first assumed that he hadn't held the tube correctly, but then, when he switched to his left eye again, he still could not see anything. Switching back and forth, he began to realize that his left eye vision was terrible. He blinked a few times, trying to clear it up. Then, without the kaleidoscope, he looked out the window, first covering one eye and then the other. He confirmed that he could see almost nothing out of his left eye. Not wishing to spoil the time with his grandson, he said nothing about it. Later that afternoon, he mentioned to his wife, "You know, honey, when Mackie and I were playing with that new toy of his, I noticed that my eyesight in the left eye is not very good."

"Why don't you get it looked at tomorrow?" she said, unalarmed. He had not told her how bad the vision really was. That evening, they watched television, and with both eyes open, he could see fine as always.

He was able to get an appointment at the Manhattan Eye and Ear Infirmary two days later. An eye resident saw him and made the diagnosis of retinal detachment, which was confirmed by the supervising faculty, an elderly retired Manhattan ophthalmologist who was volunteering for teaching duty.

"So how do I get this fixed?" Alan wanted to know. "Where should I go? Do you do that operation here?"

"Yes, we do, but if I were you, I'd go to Boston. There is this new doctor from Europe who is having a lot of success. He does this new procedure called scleral buckling. I've heard him speak about it. It's a breakthrough. We can call his office and make an appointment."

When Mr. Peszinski arrived in Boston, I was the fellow that was assigned to him. He told me that nothing had changed since he first noticed his visual problem. He was a good candidate for surgery since he was not taking any medications, other than aspirin and vitamins. The anesthetic risk would be minimal. I quickly listened to his heart and lungs and took his blood pressure—136/76, normal for his age. His pulse was 70. I asked him to lie down on the exam table, pushed on his abdomen, and felt for the edge of his liver. Everything was normal. With the patient thus supine, I adjusted the ophthalmoscope on my head, placed the drawing clipboard on his chest, got out my colored pencils, and started the retina exam and drawing, having the focusing lens in one hand and the blue-red pencil in the other. This was what we fellows were learning to do—looking very carefully at every part of the retinal detail.

At five o'clock that afternoon, Mr. Peszinski, together with the other fifteen patients to be operated the next day, gathered in the retina clinic, together with all the fellows and our faculty. One room was equipped with eight exam tables with indirect ophthalmoscopes hanging on the walls at the head of each table. The patients were lying down with clipboard on chest, and faculty would check each retina drawing meticulously. This was prime teaching time, as the drawings were refined, while teacher and student looked into the eye, one after the other. That night, Mr. Peszinski stayed overnight in the hospital, as was customary in those days, and was operated the next morning.

The surgery was uncomplicated, and the retina was reattached. I was the assistant and was able, during the procedure, to look into the eye multiple times as the retina settled down into its proper position in response to our manipulations. The surgery lasted only one and a half hours. It turned out to be the easiest case of the day. During the next two days of hospitalization, the retina remained attached, and we were able to discharge the patient a day early.

Two weeks later, the patient took the train from New York to Boston. His vision in the operated eye was still blurry, but he had no trouble coming by himself, even managing the Boston subway system to get from Back Bay to Charles Street.

Miss O'Brien checked the vision: light perception. It was really too early to expect any improvement at this time. Although I did not see the patient at this time, another fellow told me, "The back of his eye looks great."

Six weeks later, he was scheduled for another follow-up exam. Because the associate who had operated was at a medical meeting giving a lecture, another associate took his place. The vision was still light perception only. The retina looked perfectly flat without any central scarring or puckering. He asked Miss O'Brien to check the vision again. "Use some plus and minus lenses. See if you can improve it." She tried without success. He looked into the eye again. There, in the middle of the retina, where the optic nerve enters the back of the eye, it looked white, very white, like an aspirin lying in the middle of a red sheet. He immediately recognized that the patient had severe optic atrophy and that his vision would never improve because the optic nerve was severely damaged. He looked through the chart and found the medical history. The patient had never noticed his poor vision until he looked through the kaleidoscope.

"Mr. Peszinski, how long do you think your vision could have been bad before that?"

"I don't know. I'm not sure. Don't you think I would have noticed it?" was the answer.

"Maybe not. We have all seen patients who first realize they can't see when they try to look through the sight of a gun at hunting season. Every fall, we seem to have at least one patient who swears that he could see fine until he tried to go hunting. I think that you have been blind in that eye for quite a long time. No optic nerve looks that pale until it has not worked for at least many months or even years. I'm afraid that you are not going to get much vision back. You may just get a little, because your retina is reattached. We shall keep our fingers crossed."

We continued to see Mr. Peszinski ever six months. His vision never improved. He apparently resumed his life with little interruption or sense of handicap, which pleased him. It seemed as if he felt sorry for his doctors that they did not get the visual result they wanted, even though they had done a perfect job. As I thought about him, I wondered how it was even possible that all these doctors, first in New York and then in Boston, the best of the best, and their students, including me, had never noticed the optic atrophy—the white aspirin-like optic nerve in the middle of the reddish retina. It should have been obvious had we not been so focused on something we could fix. Were we stuck in a routine?

Chapter 3

Is this Research or What?

Macular edema is the most common cause of central visual loss in diabetes. It is swelling of the central retina, the macula, caused by leaking of fluid from the blood flowing through sick small macular capillaries into surrounding tissues. Diabetes, which is caused by problems of sugar metabolism, is really a vascular disease. The swelling of the macula interferes with normal function, so light coming through the optics of the eye (cornea and lens) is unable to be imaged properly and is thus transmitted as a blurred picture to the brain.

Treatments for macular edema continue to be unsatisfactory, so prevention is critical. If diabetes, especially the type II adult-onset variety, were controlled through diet, weight loss, and exercise, macular edema might never occur. In reality, however, macular edema is very common.

Around 1970, the argon laser came into use and quickly became a favorite tool to treat all sorts of eye conditions, especially in the retina. The laser beam was small, hot, and green in color and was therefore maximally absorbed by pigmented, especially red, targets. It could thus be aimed at red vascular structures in the retina and burn without doing too much collateral damage of the surrounding tissue. This was perfect for the destruction of vascular anomalies or tumors and also could be used to seal leaks in blood vessel walls. Fluorescein angiography, invented years before, made it possible to find these leaks, which could then be targeted by the argon beam.

It did not take long for retina specialists to try laser treatment for diabetic macular edema, even though not all patients showed specific leaks and some maculas were so thickened and opaque that leaks could not be identified at all. But as is so often the case in medicine, if you give a surgeon a new tool, it may well be tried before guidelines for its use have been established.

I, too, was fascinated by the laser's potential and was eager to try it. After successfully treating several patients with small vascular tumors, I was ready to attack the macula, recognizing fully well that a stray burn in the center of the macula, the fovea centralis, would lead to permanent central vision loss.

I found the perfect patient, Asrah Kababian—a short, stocky, slightly overweight rug dealer of Armenian descent. He had diabetic macular edema, which had not responded to diet and exercise despite his reasonably well-controlled diabetes. His macular edema also did not fluctuate, as it does in so many patients, and thus his vision was always around 20/200 in each eye. I had been seeing him every three months for about two years, and he and I were both tired of the lack of improvement, even though he had now lost ten pounds, was exercising, and had tried several medications which promote dehydration.

In January, he arrived for his postholiday appointment, and his vision was again 20/200 in each eye. The big *E* on the eye chart was all he could see with the best possible glasses. His central retinas looked grey and opalescent, and the angiography did not demonstrate specific leaks, just a diffused fluorescence of the intravenously injected dye, twenty minutes after injection. Would this be the patient who could show me that laser could be beneficial even before its precise mechanism of action would be understood?

I told him about the laser and how it worked to eradicate specific red leaks. Then, I told him that his situation was slightly different, because no specific leaks could be identified, although I knew they were there.

"There are several retina specialists who have tried very light laser in a grid pattern around the center of the macula in patients like you. There's especially one doctor at Johns Hopkins who strongly believes in this treatment, but he agrees that some sort of study has to be done to prove it. But meanwhile, we, in academic medicine, all need to try this and get some anecdotal data, which are needed to get the funding agencies, such as NIH, even interested in supporting a clinical trial. Are you interested?"

"I'll try anything as long as it won't damage my sight even more."

"No, I think it is fairly safe, because the laser burns that I will use are very light. In fact, they will be almost invisible to me as I am doing the procedure."

The next day, Asrah came for his treatment. I sat him down in front of the laser, went through the same explanation again, and then asked him to sign permission to do this experimental procedure. I was excited to perform it. After all, wasn't this our obligation, especially in academic medicine, to try new things? Then, if it succeeded, and if other treatments on other patients succeeded as well, we could present our small series at the next national research meeting. Then, if other investigators had similar results, we might have enough anecdotal evidence to instigate interest in starting the national prospective controlled clinical trial, hopefully funded by NIH, in which we could participate. I had enough time before the March deadline to put a presentation together for the May research meeting.

The procedure was not difficult to perform. Even though both eyes looked similar, I flipped a coin to remove any bias about which eye to treat. Tails meant the left eye. Then, as had been suggested by my Hopkins colleague, I placed a tiny two-hundred micron burn in the peripheral retina, where there was no edema, so that I could gauge what strength burn to use if I were treating a red lesion. Then, I cut the power by 50 percent and placed a grid (nine-by-nine burn square with burns two hundred microns apart) in the swollen macular region. It was slightly scary, since the burns were barely visible, and

I had little idea of how much of the energy would be absorbed and at what level within the retina. It took all of five minutes, and the patient held perfectly still and felt nothing.

"Is that it?" he asked.

"That's all there is to it. Now, let's see if it works."

Asrah put his hand on his right eye, nodded, and said, "Well, I can still see the same as before."

"Please come to see me again in about ten days. Call me if there is a change. Here's my private phone number. I'm really anxious to know what happens."

Ten days later, he appeared on my schedule again. I had not heard from him. It was my morning to work with a resident-in-training and have a medical student observe what ophthalmology was all about. The resident spent about ten minutes with each patient, taking the interim history, testing the best-corrected vision, taking the eye pressure, and instilling the dilating drops to facilitate the retina exam. When he was finished with Asrah, he turned on the yellow light in the hallway above the exam room door, which would automatically turn green ten minutes later, indicating that the patient was ready to be seen by me, with pupils dilated.

When the medical student and I came into the room, the resident was already there. He looked up from the chart and immediately said, "There's quite an improvement in Mr. Kababian's vision—20/40 in the right and still 20/200 in the left. Amazing!"

I was elated.

"Go ahead and take a look at the macula and tell me what you see."

The resident was delighted to take the first look. He saw it as a compliment that his teacher would listen to his judgment, and it was testimony to his examination skills. He looked intensely at the improved macula and then switched the examination contact lens to the other eye for comparison. Meanwhile, the medical student, standing between the desk and me, was perusing the chart.

"I don't see much difference between the two eyes," said the resident, "but perhaps the right eye has slightly less edema in the macula. Certainly, it seems less grey, less opalescent. I see no laser burns anywhere."

"Let me take a look."

He and I switched places while I asked, "Asrah, do you think you can see better?" "Today, I think I can, but a couple of days ago, it was just like before."

"Maybe it just takes a few days for the laser burns to scar down. That would be what I would expect. Usually, these burns get absorbed either by red structures such as retinal blood vessels or else by the RPE, the pigment layer directly under the retina, which has a lot to do with keeping the retina dry, dehydrated, and thin, not swollen with edema. It would seem quite normal for a burn to take even up to ten days to become a scar. We don't really know how such scars really work, but certainly we know that some scarring can thin out a thickened retina." The medical student was listening intently.

As I duplicated the resident's exam, I had to agree that in the right eye, the edema was less than before, and there was no visible evidence of laser burns. I pushed back from the slit-lamp microscope.

"All this is very interesting. I am not sure what we have learned. I sure don't know how this happened, I don't know the mechanism of action, but I do know that this kind of light laser can make a difference, can sometimes improve vision. I wonder if we should present this case at some meeting or even publish it."

As I leaned back away from the patient and looked up at the standing resident, I noticed that the medical student was pointing at the chart. He was mumbling something to the resident, who was nodding affirmatively.

"What is it?" I asked.

"Excuse me, Dr. van Heuven, but this student just noticed something. It says here that you treated the left eye, but—let me double-check—yes, it is the right eye which improved. Is that right?"

I quickly pulled the chart from the desk and found the treatment page.

"My god, guys, you are right, absolutely right. How is this possible? How embarrassing! I guess that the laser has done nothing!

The improvement in the other eye must have been due to a fluctuation in the edema, which happens all the time in some patients."

I now turned fully toward the medical student, stretching out my hand to shake his. "I guess it takes a medical student to teach a professor something about nonscientific wishful thinking. I guess we are all learning something today."

Later on, at the May national research meeting, one of the residents and I presented a short paper on diplopia (double vision) in glaucoma patients, totally unrelated to macular edema. We probably should have told this story instead.

Postscript

During the 1980s, the NIH sponsored a multicenter prospective controlled clinical trial on the laser treatment of diabetic macular edema, which was able to prove its efficacy in a select group of patients.

Part III

KEEP YOUR EYES OPEN

Chapter 1: The Fiancé 67
Chapter 2: The Turtleneck 73
Chapter 3: White Spots 79
Chapter 4: Deviation 86
Chapter 5: Black Spots 97

Chapter 1

THE FIANCÉ

Our maid Henny had been a member of our family for many years, ever since age seventeen. At that time, she had just graduated from high school in a neighboring village and came to us as a mother's helper when our children were two and five. She lived under the eaves of an attic room, which had previously been used for storage but was now freshly painted in yellow and white, with two skylights, which provided much cheeriness. She was an open-faced youthful blonde of Northern European extraction, appearing younger than her age except for her rimless glasses, was orderly and conservative, and was a constant and reliable presence in our family. She was almost like an older daughter, but she intuitively respected the unspoken line that was drawn between family and servant. She participated in almost everything we did and traveled with us when we vacationed in Mexico, Switzerland, or Nantucket. I don't ever remember taking a vacation without her. Her daily routine consisted of childcare, cleaning, cooking, and spending much time in the kitchen, which was her living room and where she had her meals. Our children loved and trusted her and were surprised to hear, after seven years, that she was leaving us to go back home, because she now had a boyfriend from her village, whom she had met during one of her free weekends when she would take the bus home to visit her parents. If she lived back at home, she thought that she could see him more often. When she moved out, she promised to return once a week as a cleaning lady.

The boyfriend, Alex, was the same one we had already met when he had come in his pick-up truck on a couple of Sunday mornings to take Henny to the Catholic church. He was a comfortable thirty-year-old, soft-spoken, and the only son of a farmer, who had died in his thirties as a result of a bizarre accident—falling off a hay wagon. When his mother remarried and had five more children, all daughters, he took on the role of helping to take care of the young girls, which stimulated his early maturity. His neatly combed russet hair and pale reddish-blotchy freckled face bespoke sensitivity to sunlight. No wonder he always wore a baseball cap when he went outside, although he politely removed it as soon as he saw us. The skin of his hands was similarly affected, and he always had multiple Band-Aids around his fingers. I knew that his trade was cabinetry, which he did indoors, so working with tools might have caused the damage to his hands, although it seemed odd that a professional cabinetmaker would injure himself so often.

Henny came every Thursday with the early bus and was already busy cleaning the house by 8:00 AM. Between four and five o'clock, Alex would arrive to pick her up and take her home. Sometimes she wasn't quite finished, so he would sit in the kitchen and pour himself some tea, which was always available. One Thursday, my surgical day, two of my cases were cancelled, and I came home early. Alex had just arrived, so I sat down with him on the small kitchen patio for a cup of tea. He boiled the water and poured it into our mugs, into which we dipped the tea bags. I tried to take a sip, but the mug was too hot to hold. Alex, however, whose fingers still had multiple Band-Aids, picked up his mug, blew onto the surface, and carefully slurped some hot liquid. "Too hot," he said, but he continued to hold on to the cup. Later, when I thought about this episode, I wondered what made his hands so insensitive. Had he damaged his hands so much during his carpentry?

We had a nice conversation. He hoped that Henny and he would get engaged pretty soon so that they could marry in the fall. He

THE EYE: WINDOW TO BODY AND SOUL

was making enough money with his woodworking, and she could continue to clean for us and perhaps for some others as well. He now needed to get more things out of the way to get ready. He was painting his house and remodeling the bathroom. He also wanted to make sure that Henny and he were both healthy, though they really had no complaints. I suggested that he also have his eyes tested, which I had already done for Henny. She was fine, just a little nearsighted, but her corrected vision was 20/20. "Maybe glasses would help you as well so you don't keep banging up your hands," I joked as I pointed at the Band-Aids. He smiled.

I saw him in the office the following week. His vision was excellent both at distance and close-up. Since he had never seen an ophthalmologist before, I performed a complete exam and dilated his pupils, warning him that he might have some trouble doing carpentry for the rest of the day, since the drops would paralyze his focusing ability.

"I'll cut my fingers even worse," he joked. For a moment, the remark caught my attention, but then I continued my exam. Both eyes looked normal. When I reclined the exam chair for the peripheral retinal exam, I did notice a small red spot in one eye and initially paid little attention to it. The whole retina looked very red, quite normal for a pale redhead, and small normal vascular twists and turns can often mimic red spots when, in fact, they are merely variations of normal. Looking at the other eye, I noticed two more red bumps, one of which was slightly larger, at least three times the width of a normal blood vessel. I looked back at the first eye and realized that these red spots were indeed abnormalities, small to be sure, no more than one millimeter in diameter, that might represent tiny vascular tumors. Each one had two blood vessels going into it, presumably an arteriole and a venule, one to feed it and one to drain it. Especially in the case of the largest tumor, these vessels were thicker than other vessels in the retina. I wondered if these were early but typical von Hippel tumors, although I had never seen them so small before. Usually such hemangioblastomas never came to an eye doctor until they were the size of a small pea and had already leaked serum or blood into the eye, causing visual symptoms. As I stepped back to talk to Alex, my headlamp's light grazed his hands, which were folded on his stomach. Was all this related—his damaged hands and his eye tumors?

"You have a few small abnormalities, some unusual blood vessels, in both eyes," I said. "It's not a big deal, and it's causing no problems. But let me ask you about some other things."

He was now sitting up. I reached over to touch one of his hands. "Can you feel this?"

"Well, I know you are touching my hand."

"Now, close your eyes for a minute and say yes as soon as you feel me scratching the back of your hand."

He complied but said nothing as I moved my black pencil over his knuckles. He also did not respond as I stroked the thin skin on the back of his hand. When he opened his eyes and looked down, he said, "Now you are stroking my hand."

"But can you really feel it?" I asked.

"I guess not. My hands are pretty tough."

During the next twenty minutes, we determined that his numbness extended to his arms as well. Now, suspecting that Alex might have similar vascular abnormalities elsewhere in his nervous system, I recommended that he also see another doctor—a friend of mine, Arthur Kuyck, a neurosurgeon—to find out more about his numbness. "I think the reason why you keep injuring your hands is that they are really numb. You can't feel it when you scrape or cut or burn yourself. That needs to be fixed, if possible. Don't you agree?"

A week later, Arthur Kuyck called me. The neurological exam had demonstrated an extensive loss of feeling in all four extremities. In addition, there was unequivocal muscular weakness in Alex's right leg. Vascular imaging studies had been done, which confirmed several separate vascular tumors in his spinal cord, apparently compressing the nerve tracts. This was thus a case of von Hippel-Lindau disease, vascular tumors in the nervous system as well as the retina. Dr. Kuyck recommended surgery to remove the tumors, even though they were probably not cancerous. They were simply in a bad location, compressing vital structures.

During the next few weeks, Alex became my patient. First, using an argon laser, I was able to burn and totally destroy the retinal tumors. Although knowing that other new tumors might appear in the future, it made sense to get rid of them before they caused visual problems. The ease by which this outpatient laser procedure was performed, without any discomfort to the patient, seemed to give Alex much-needed confidence in the next neurosurgical procedure. Henny, now that she lived near him, also helped greatly, taking much of the stress out of the situation, using a remarkable combination of sober pragmatism and genuine love.

The spinal surgery was extensive and long because of three different tumor locations. It successfully removed all tumors without causing additional spinal cord injury, thanks to Kuyck's expertise.

The recovery was slow, with considerable back pain, but was nonetheless accelerated by frequent physical therapy. A few months later, Alex and Henny became engaged. After the winter, now after almost a year of delay, they planned their wedding. Their lives had resumed a normal schedule except for the periodic checkups with Kuyck and with me. This was the time when I had several discussions with Henny concerning the dominant inheritance pattern of von Hippel-Lindau syndrome. She repeatedly asserted that they were not ready for children anyway until she knew that he was totally cured. This was not the answer I sought.

The wedding was an intimate family affair, conservative Catholic, according to tradition. My wife and I attended as two of only a small group of friends, the others all being related one way or another to Henny's and Alex's parents and their five and nine siblings each. These were still the days of large Catholic families. After the ceremony, I noticed that Alex had no bandages on his fingers. Later, he informed me that some of the sensation in his hands and arms had actually returned, and he could now work better without injuring himself.

For two years, Alex was medically stable. During that time, I saw him every six months, as did Kuyck. He was also being followed by a general practitioner, whose task was, knowing the propensity of von Hippel-Lindau patients to develop tumors or even cancer elsewhere, to check his general health. Then, Alex developed some back pain. At first, the GP ascribed it to the spinal surgery, "which could give you some arthritis later." After three months of painkillers, he finally called Kuyck, who recommended kidney function studies immediately and said he would see him right away.

The neurologic exam actually showed improvement. Not only had his sensation in his limbs improved, but the strength of his two legs was now almost equal. The kidney function tests, however, were borderline normal, and the urine demonstrated the presence of a few blood cells. X-rays were done with and without contrast. It was now certain that Alex had a kidney tumor. A few days later, a urologic surgeon removed it. It was malignant and had already invaded neighboring tissues. Not all of it was surgically resectable. Radiation and some chemotherapy were of no help. A miserable, painful six months ensued. Then, Alex died of metastatic kidney cancer, which had spread to his brain. An autopsy revealed not only that brain tumor but also another hemangioma, the size of a walnut, in his cerebellum, at the base of the brain—another part of the von Hippel-Lindau syndrome.

After a few months, Henny moved back in with us and again became part of the family routine, taking her place at the kitchen table and sleeping under the eaves, as if nothing had ever happened.

PS: Von Hippel-Lindau Syndrome is a dominantly inherited combination of retinal hemangiomas (von Hippel) and central nervous system hemangiomas, often in the cerebellum or spinal cord (Lindau). Because of the constant threat of recurrence, close follow-up is recommended. Due to the presence of a variety of kidney problems, early renal studies are suggested. Because of the dominant genetic pattern, a family history and the examination of family members is important as well as genetic counseling.

Chapter 2

THE TURTLENECK

I was not surprised to hear about her athletic endeavors. She had run several marathons—the easiest in Phoenix because it was flat and without humidity, but the most exciting one in New York City over the Verrazano Bridge. Then, because of leg cramps, she had to take up bicycling instead and was doing one hundred miles per week on a hybrid bike, which she could use for longer trips as well. She was also on a mission to climb the tallest peak in every American state and had already managed to do so in thirty-two of the fifty. She looked and moved like an athlete, with a lively spring in her step and a perky manner. She was dressed in a sporty turtleneck shirt with long sleeves, capri pants, and white running shoes. Although only thirty-eight years old, she had gray hair, which she kept boyishly short, cropped to keep it out of her eyes.

The reason for her office visit was a sudden decrease in vision in her left eye. Because she was an emergency room nurse from our own hospital, we got her an immediate appointment—the day after it happened. Our technician took her history. She had no medical issues and prided herself on her excellent physical condition. The only problems had been related to sports. She once broke an ankle many years ago while sliding down a snowy slope on her descent from Mt. Rainier. She told the tale of the splint she had to fashion out of a tree branch in order to make it down the mountain. And oh yes, she once had a stomach bleed in her early twenties, probably an ulcer from the stress of nursing school, but that never recurred. She did not know much about her family history, partly because her father died of a heart attack in his late twenties during a football game. He played for the Dallas Cowboys. It had been quite a story. "It was in all the papers." Her mother was still alive, had remarried after many years, and was very healthy. She had no siblings.

The sudden vision problem in one eye occurred while biking. A truck had passed her, and something had flown out of the truck into her eye. "Probably some dirt." She had blinked it out and rubbed her eye quite hard. Then, it felt better, but the vision was blurry. It did not improve over the next few hours. The problem seemed to be in the center of her vision.

"I can see just fine on the sides, but there is just this blockage right in the middle," she emphasized, using her hands to illustrate.

The tech did the preliminary exam. The vision was 20/30 with the right, but 20/400 with the left eye. No improvement was possible with refraction. The front of both eyes looked normal, and the pupils constricted normally in response to bright light. I saw her after dilation. The retina exam gave the answer. There was a large two-by-three-millimeter roundish hemorrhage in the retina centrally, clearly the cause of her symptom.

"You have a small bleed in your macula," I said, "right smack in the center of your retina. You got this how?"

She recounted the story of something flying into her eye while biking.

"How hard did that hit you?" I asked, not observing any external evidence of trauma—no skin bruise or conjunctival redness.

"I don't think very hard. It wasn't large, just some dirt. I rubbed it out!"

"How hard did you rub it?" "Oh, I don't know."

"I hear you are quite an athlete. Have you done anything very strenuous to make this happen, like lifting weights? Do you ever lift weights while you are lying down?"

"No, I don't, no." Her answer was thoughtfully slow.

"How about straining while your head is down, like sit-ups, or even hanging upside down from these boots that some people have? Do you do any of that? We call that type of straining a Valsalva maneuver. I'm sure you have heard of it in nursing school. It really increases the blood pressure in your head."

"Sometimes I do sit-ups, but not recently." "You don't play the trumpet, do you?"

She smiled. "No, that's for sure." Then she added with a short chuckle, "I guess sometimes I like to blow my own horn."

I looked again at the retina. The small central blood clot was under and also in the retina, thus blocking light from reaching the more deeply located rod and cone receptors. The blood was dark red, like a clot, surrounded by the orange color of the normal background. However, there was something peculiar in the orange appearance just adjacent to the hemorrhage, which caught my attention. It looked mottled, like splattered paint. I had only seen this once before in a patient with angioid streaks, which this patient did not have. Such streaks, which appear like an extra set of blood vessels radiating out from the optic nerve, are linear pigment disturbances actually located under the retina. They represent cracks in the elastic layer of the eye. Such cracks are areas of fragility and can occasionally lead to bleeding, even from minor trauma.

As I was thinking, I looked back at the patient. Although it was July, I wondered about her turtleneck shirt. Why would she wear something so warm when the weather was already eighty degrees? Was she hiding something?

"Excuse me for asking," I said. "Do you always wear turtlenecks?"
"Yes, most of the time. It's easy when you do sports."

"Would you mind pulling your collar down a bit so I can look at your neck?" She raised her eyebrows but obliged. The skin at the base of her neck was grayish brown, darker than the color of her face and hands, and was finely wrinkled, like the aging skin of a much older person.

"I've always had a funny-looking neck," she said. "The kids in school called me chicken skin, so I started wearing turtlenecks to cover it up. Children can be so cruel to one another, especially girls. Later in high school, after I became captain of the hockey team, they stopped messing with me. In fact, they all started wearing turtlenecks. It became a fad." She pulled up her right sleeve. "See, I have the same thing on my arms, but other than the funny appearance, it doesn't bother me."

It was now becoming more obvious to me why she had the macular hemorrhage. Her history of the stomach bleed, the leg cramps, the skin changes, and the macular hemorrhage were all pointing to the same diagnosis. The mottled orange appearance probably represented what the textbooks call peau d'orange, looking like the skin of an orange. This patient had PXE, pseudoxanthoma elasticum, and she probably inherited it from her father, who had coronary artery disease from the same cause. That might have caused his heart attack at an early age.

"Now I think I know why you had this bleeding in your eye," I told her. "It was probably the same reason that you had that gastrointestinal hemorrhage years ago." I went on to explain PXE as a disease of elastic tissue, sometimes dominantly inherited and causing problems with parts of the body, where elastic tissue is of critical importance. Blood vessels are affected by early calcification, which could compromise circulation to the limbs and heart and even to the brain. It could also cause gastrointestinal bleeds, usually from the stomach.

"Most patients have skin wrinkling, just like you have on your neck, inside your elbows, and probably around your belly button." She nodded affirmatively. "You know," I continued, "your leg cramps may have been due to the same thing—not enough blood going to your legs when you really stressed those muscles while running. In your eye, PXE really makes the wall of your eye very fragile, and even a moderate rubbing of your eye, like you did to get the dirt out, could have caused the bleeding. However, this blood will clear up, and I predict that your vision will improve again and even become normal. You know, blood disintegrates and will get absorbed. You'll be fine with your vision. Just stop rubbing your eye."

I was fully aware that my optimism was risky, because I knew of many instances where the clot of such a retinal hemorrhage resulted in a macular scar with permanent poor vision, but the patient seemed to need some good news. Also, I really could not see any angioid streaks, and the patients who had developed macular scars all had very visible and large streaks running through the macula.

I continued to explain, "Look upon this as a lucky moment in your life." I smiled. "God has just given you a little warning, a little suggestion to be especially careful, because you have a minor genetic problem. You know that you are pretty healthy and in great shape, much better than most people your age, and that you can do almost anything physically. But in your case, you need to check certain aspects of your health on a regular basis so that any little PXE-related issue can be dealt with before it causes any problems. Meanwhile, keep living your normal life and stay in shape!"

That morning, after an exam, fluorescein angiography of both eyes was performed, which faintly demonstrated angioid streaks bilaterally. I showed her the pictures and explained the importance of protecting the eyes from minor injuries, especially during sports. I recommended sports goggles and instructed the desk clerk to give her the information about where to obtain them. Since she was approaching forty and had mentioned some difficulty reading tiny print, I suggested not just reading glasses, but bifocals, which would also correct her mild myopia at distance while protecting her eyes.

"You can wear these all day long while you're working," I encouraged her. "I bet you'll also see better while you're driving."

By the time she departed, she had appointments scheduled with a cardiovascular specialist, a gastroenterologist, and a dermatologist. During the next few weeks, she had blood work done, including special tests for calcium and phosphorous metabolism. Her skin biopsy confirmed the PXE diagnosis, and the EKG stress test and GI series were all normal. She returned to see me as the hemorrhage slowly cleared. At three months, her vision was 20/70, and six months later, it had returned to 20/30. Her bifocals improved her to 20/20 in each eye.

She was happy and unconcerned, accepting a life of regular doctor visits while maintaining her athletic habits. Her regular schedule now included yearly visits to my office for fluorescein angiography to detect early small recurrences as well as regular gastrointestinal endoscopy and cardiovascular ultrasound and stress tests. Twice, during the next ten years, I had to perform laser treatment of small vascular leaks under the retina. Then, at age forty-nine, she underwent a stent placement in one of her coronary arteries, but none of it ever slowed her down, especially since she was never symptomatic. The last time I saw her, she looked fine, ready to move back to Pennsylvania to become the nursing director of the Surgical Intensive Care Unit at Lancaster Hospital.

Chapter 3

WHITE SPOTS

Great teachers are great liars because they simplify. They create a black-and-white universe, which, in reality, is in Technicolor. This effective means of teaching superimposes rules on the world that are best learned before the exceptions to those rules should be taught. The words *always* and *never*, favorites of good teachers, do not describe reality very well, especially in the complex fields of biology and medicine. In medicine, *always* is never the case and *never* is always wrong.

In medical school, we learned that right lower quadrant abdominal pain with rebound tenderness (pain when the doctor suddenly releases pressure on the abdomen) means acute appendicitis. Then we add "unless proven otherwise," which happens at least 25 percent of the time and means that the rule is wrong one out of four times. Still the rule is important to know. In ophthalmology, too, we have rules. For example, white spots in or under retina are always significant and should always be explored and explained.

One type of white spot, a soft exudate of the retina, is really a tiny area of edema (swelling) due to the closure of a small capillary, rending the normally transparent retina opaque, like a pearl. Normally, the inside back of the eye, the so-called fundus, looks red, because of a layer of red blood vessels under the transparent retina. That is the choroid layer, which provides much of the blood supply to the retina. Thus, when a small area of retina turns from transparent to white, it really stands out against the red background and, although tiny, is hard to miss with an ophthalmoscope.

Soft exudates, also known as cotton-wool spots, always demand an explanation—that is the rule. What would make a small capillary want to become obstructed? Is it due to an arterial spasm, such as may occur in hypertension or migraine, or is it an embolus, a piece of calcium or cholesterol coming from elsewhere, such as a heart valve or a carotid artery? Possibly it is due to a local disease of the capillary wall, such as may occur in diabetes or a variety of autoimmune diseases in which vasculitis occurs, an inflammation of the blood vessel wall. Then it might also be due to some blood disorder, which either increases the viscosity of blood or interferes with the normal blood-clotting mechanism. There are many possibilities.

I particularly remember one patient, a thirty-four-year-old beautiful, athletic-looking woman with long straight dark-brown hair framing her tanned face. Her green-gray eyes, like those of a husky dog, accentuated her fine features: thin, straight nose; high cheekbones; and delicate chin. With little movement of her thin lips as she spoke, you could see her perfectly straight and very white upper teeth, to which some dentist must have paid considerable attention. She reminded me of an Argentinian film star. She spoke precisely with emphasis on *s* and *t* sounds, never slurring a word, and with the slightest hint of a Spanish accent. She had been born in the United Sates, but her father was from Peru. Her name was Maria Calderon. The patient list indicated "blurred vision while reading" as the chief complaint. Mentally, that prepared me for a quick visit, probably resulting in a prescription for reading glasses.

Her history was, as expected, uncomplicated. She was single but engaged to be married to an economics professor at Trinity University. Her career drive had resulted in a vice president position at the regional Seabrook Bank, and now she was aiming to start a family with, she insisted, no more than two children. Like many in her generation, she exercised daily. Yoga was too calm for her, but jogging was her sport, running a faithful fifty miles every week with two one-day breaks in the routine and no less than fifteen miles on Saturdays, at a comfortable 7–1/2 mile-per-hour pace. Most weekends, she would try to sign up for a race, but so many of them were ten kilometers or less that she preferred to do the fifteen miles on her own. She had no significant health problems other than a rare cold and took no medications. The frequent tingling in her feet was clearly due to the jogging, as was her sporadic dizziness, which she ascribed to dehydration from running on hot days. The migraine headaches, which she had as a pubescent girl, were now less frequent. Her other headaches, she laughed, were all stress-related, often before board meetings with "all those male chauvinistic egos" at the bank.

"I'm sure they all wonder why there is even a female on the board."

"Have you ever had any kind of surgery?" I wanted to know.

"Well, yes. I broke my ankle once skiing many years ago. Now, I can't remember, really, which leg it was."

"Any eye problems or ear problems?"

"No, except recently. Sometimes, I can't see to read. I have to blink my eyes and then hold things farther away from me so that I don't, like, see double, or something."

"Have you ever had glasses?" "No."

"Have you ever seen any eye doctors before?"

"No, except many, many years ago, we all, as students, had our eyes checked by the school when I was in in first or second grade. I think that they brought in an optometrist to do that. He tried to give me glasses, but I never got them. I would always see just fine."

The eye exam proceeded quickly, as we were talking. Her vision was 20/15 at distance and 20/25 at near, suggesting some loss of focusing ability. At her age of thirty-four, that seemed premature, unless she had been farsighted all along, meaning that her eyes' optical system (cornea and lens) were not strong enough to muster the additional optical power to focus on near objects. If she had not been farsighted, probably since birth, she would not get such symptoms until she was about forty or later.

To diagnose farsightedness in this young person, the pupils needed to be dilated to paralyze the focusing muscle. Since this was her first ophthalmic visit, it was also important to examine the lens and the structures in the back of the eyes, the retinas, the blood vessels, and the optic nerves.

Twenty minutes following the eye drops, I was able to confirm her slight farsightedness (hyperopia), which "we can fix with reading glasses. Just put them on at work when you want to read or look at the computer. Get the narrow ones so that you can look over the top at things farther away. There's no need to wear glasses when you drive or walk around. You can even get more than one pair so you can have one at the office and another one at home by your computer."

The rest of the eye exam was pretty normal. The pupils dilated well, the lenses were clear, and the optic nerves appeared normal. The retinas were shiny, normal for a young person, and the maculas were entirely normal. Just nasal to the optic nerve was a small whitish-gray fuzzy area, no more than one millimeter in diameter, which I, at first, overlooked since I was not expecting to find any abnormalities. But then, at my second perusal of the fundus, I recognized either a cotton-wool spot or else an area of myelinated nerve fibers, with which she would have been born with. The latter is a congenital abnormality where some myelin, a whitish substance normally present as a sheath along peripheral nerves, is accidentally deposited, during fetal development, along some retinal nerves. Myelin, in that location, is of no clinical significance and can appear similar to a cotton-wool spot. Both are whitish, and both are surface phenomena. Since the patient was so healthy, I immediately favored the myelin diagnosis, and I told her about it. I then cleaned my exam lens and my fingers, which were now covered with makeup. As I walked her back to the front desk to check out, I asked her who her boss was at the bank.

"What's the name of the president? I think I know him."

It's . . . uh, it's ah . . . this is crazy, I just can't think of it right now. My office is right next to his. I'm blocking it . . . so odd." She shook her head.

As we approached the desk, I interrupted her, "Why don't we take a picture of that white spot, now that you're dilated? Then, I'll give you a copy, just in case you ever see another eye doctor. You can pull this out and show him that it has been there for a while."

After the photo, she walked out of the office with an energetic spring in her step, as if ready to start jogging.

The following week, a copy of the fundus photo appeared on my office computer. Now it was obvious that the white spot was indeed a soft exudate—a cotton-wool spot, a miniature area of ischemic retinal edema indicating a small vascular occlusion.

Maria was surprised to hear from me when I telephoned and told her to come back for another visit. At that time, I would examine her retina again and also order some blood tests, which could be done at the local lab.

"Do I really need all this?" she asked. "I really feel fine, and I am quite busy."

Trying not to alarm her, I told her that I would be remiss not to pursue the cause of the white spot.

"But it's probably nothing. Let's just make sure." Then, jokingly, I said, "You'll have to forgive me for being thorough." She laughed.

When she returned two days later, she wanted to get it over with. She was late for her appointment. She had already called the front desk that morning to find out exactly when the appointment was, because she had forgotten. Then, when she appeared at 11:00 AM for her 9:00 AM appointment, she said, "I'm sure you told me eleven o'clock. I didn't write it down, but that's what I heard." And then, shaking her head, she added, "I'm always forgetting things."

After dilating her pupils, I reexamined the retina, looking meticulously for other white areas. I also performed scleral depression, indenting the eyeball slightly with a small probe in order to visualize the far peripheral retina, which I had not done before. To my surprise, I saw numerous fine white lines radiating out. Upon further inspection, it was clear that these lines were the occluded ends of many of the small peripheral arterioles in both retinas.

I told Maria there were a couple of other little spots in her retina of both eyes and that we should definitely do the blood tests I had spoken about. And to be sure that everything was okay, she should see her regular doctor.

"I don't have a doctor," she quickly stated, shrugging her shoulders and raising her eyebrows. "Do I really need one? I feel just fine."

"Let me get you an appointment with a friend of mine, a wonderful family doctor, David Pape, who can probably fit you in real soon. How about next Wednesday? By then, I will have the results of some of the blood tests."

She reluctantly agreed but couldn't resist the comment, spoken with a smile on her face, "Aren't you just doing a bunch of unnecessary stuff? I know I am insured, but isn't this just like what people complain about, running up a huge medical bill for little reason?"

"Maria, believe me, I would never do that, but if you were my daughter, I would say, 'Do these tests and see that doctor,' because frankly, I am a little concerned about you. I don't wish to alarm you. There is probably a simple and benign explanation for all of this, but we must make sure it isn't serious."

Before she left, I took her blood pressure and pulse. Both were normal, but I noticed that her hand was cold. The lab tests I ordered were meant to exclude leukemia and other blood cell abnormalities. In addition, a sedimentation rate was done to rule out the remote possibility of temporal arteritis, which would be unlikely in a young person. A few days later, after she saw David Pape, other tests were ordered to explore blood clotting abnormalities and potential sources of emboli (pieces of calcium or cholesterol in the blood stream), which could travel to small peripheral arteries in the retina and elsewhere. Other blood tests looked for causes of vascular inflammation, and ultrasound examinations were done of the carotid arteries and heart to search for sources of emboli, even though the internist's exam was normal. He had also noticed her meticulous attention to clear speech and asked her about it. Apparently, a year before, she had experienced an episode of sudden dizziness and difficulty saying some words, particularly the *s* sound, which came out sounding more like "th."

The most significant test result was that two tests for lupus, systemic lupus erythematosus, were positive. She was also anemic. Putting that information together with her headaches, tingling of her feet, cold hands, fainting spells, dizziness, slurred speech, and forgetfulness "made the diagnosis of lupus pretty clear"—so said David Pape. I agreed and added that she wore a lot of make-up on her cheeks, probably to cover the typical "butterfly" rash, which so many lupus patients have.

Dr. Pape's excellent bedside manner and a couple of phone conversations convinced Maria that she should see both a neurologist and a cardiologist. She wanted an explanation of her memory loss, which she had now realized was very specific: names and numbers. As a banker, she was especially concerned with her difficulty with numbers. Meanwhile, he started treating her with chloroquine and cortisone. Dr. Weinstein, the neurologist, saw her two weeks later. By then, she was willing to recognize how serious her memory loss had become, and she was worried about rapid worsening. The MRI that he ordered indicated multiple small lacunar infarcts of the brain, basically evidence of small strokes. He called her with the bad news and made an appointment with a cardiologist. He recommended the addition of a blood thinner, which was started immediately.

That weekend, less than a month following my first appointment with her, Maria suffered a massive heart attack during a ten-mile footrace and died before the ambulance reached the emergency room.

Her fiancé, a charming tall lank man in his midthirties, whom I had never met before, later told me that she had been worried recently, but he did not know why. He had encouraged her to enter the race, because it always made her feel better. However, she had never mentioned lupus to him or the fact that she was seeing so many doctors. Ironically, she never made it to the cardiologist, although it seems doubtful that he could have saved her.

Much later, as I thought about this sad case, I recollected the rule about white spots in the retina: white spots are always significant. This was no exception.

Chapter 4

Deviation

The COMS (Collaborative Ocular Melanoma Study) started in the 1980s, at the strong urging of one of the leaders of ophthalmology, Dr. Bradley Straatsma, then chairman at UCLA's Jules Stein Eye Institute. There was considerable skepticism about its need because several melanoma centers, such as the ones in Boston, Philadelphia, and San Francisco, had developed their own unique best methods of treatment, and many patients with suspected eye melanoma were referred to these centers of excellence. Thus, there was the concern that not enough patients would be available to recruit for such a national study, since eye melanoma was relatively rare, with only about two thousand cases being reported each year in the United States, many of whom would be referred to these historic and outstanding centers. If there were such a national study, would ophthalmologists change their referral patterns and refer their patients to COMS centers, or would they, and their patients, continue to prefer the established centers where immediate treatment, without randomization into different treatment groups, was already available? As it turned out, the National Institutes of Health (NIH) did support and fund the COMS, established COMS centers throughout the United States, and was able to carry out a successful study with enough patients to answer some very basic questions about what and when to treat and what type of treatment should be given. For the first time, standardization was achieved in the measurement of the tumors and in the delivery of treatment. Now, data from different centers could be compared, which had never been possible before, when, for example, a small tumor in Boston might have been the same as a medium-sized tumor in Philadelphia. Also, the radiation type and dosage had been markedly different between centers, so few conclusions from published data could really be drawn about whether radiation worked or not or how well.

At the University of Texas Health Science Center in San Antonio, we were fortunate to be chosen as one of the COMS centers, so eye tumors or even suspected tumor patients were referred from a large area in the South Central United States and Mexico. One such patient, an elderly man of small proportions with a slow, careful shuffling step, slightly stooped and quietly looking down, was brought in by an energetic, athletic woman of around fifty, who seemed in charge and very comfortable in the formality of a doctor's office. Her manner at the reception desk was assertive.

"We're on time, even a few minutes early," she told the receptionist. "So how long is it going to be before we are seen?"

"As soon as the doctor is finished with the patient he's with now, madam." "Well, what do you think—five minutes, ten minutes, or what?"

"I really don't know, madam . . . but-but soon."

The fierce look and aggressive manner of the patient's daughter had intimidated the gentler, soft-spoken Hispanic desk clerk.

"Well, I'm a nurse, and I can't wait forever. We came all the way from Harlingen and want to get back before dark." She turned around and sat down after she had helped the patient sit also. "Sit down, Dad. We'll just wait." The man said nothing and continued to stare at the floor.

Twenty minutes later, I walked into the exam room, where, a few minutes earlier, the technician had installed the patient. In another screening room, she had already performed the preliminary exam: history, vision, eye pressure, pupillary reactions, a crude measure of the peripheral visual field, and blood pressure. Finding everything normal, she had then dilated the pupils with eye drops, which would take about fifteen minutes to work.

The man was sitting on the exam chair, and the woman was sitting, straight up without leaning back, in a corner chair.

"My father is here because of an eye tumor," she announced. "It was noticed by Dr. Adelsohn in Harlingen. He wasn't quite sure if it was malignant or something else, but he had never seen it before, and we have been going to him for years. So it must be something new. I'm a nurse, so I made an appointment right away. They squeezed us in within a week. That was great. I just hate to wait for an appointment when I know it could be serious. I guess, as a nurse, I know too much, and things like this worry me."

I checked the tech's notes and then started to look at the patient. He was about five feet eight inches tall and of slight build, not weighing more than 130 pounds. His health had been good except for some weakness, which had started two years before, and an irregular pulse, which I confirmed by palpating his wrist. His only medications were a blood thinner and Colace for constipation. As I pulled the slit lamp between us to begin the exam, I asked about the weakness.

"Well, he seemed to have gotten weak right after my mother died of cancer. One doctor thought that he might have had a small stroke, but I don't think so. He is just generally weak. He doesn't do much—watches some television, listens to a lot of radio. He loves public radio, especially the opera, and will sit for hours on his chair with his eyes closed, listening. I'm never sure if he is just dozing or what. When Mother died, I had an extra room downstairs, so I moved him in with me. He's an easy roommate. I go to work early and get back by four o'clock in the afternoon. I think he gets up late and has some breakfast, judging from what's left in the refrigerator, and then has the sandwich I make him for lunch. We always have dinner together. He never complains." She then added, "I never thought that living with a man could be so easy, not after my ex-husband." She chuckled.

The tumor in the right eye was of medium size, like a small pea. It was located on the nasal side of his retina and had all the characteristics of a melanoma—brown pigment and a location clearly in the choroid, the layer of blood vessels underneath the retina. Otherwise, the exam of both eyes was essentially normal, except for the barely significant cataract in both eyes, not an abnormal finding in any seventy-three-year-old person.

I started to talk to the patient about choroidal melanoma and asked him if he had ever heard of it before. He nodded yes and now spoke for the first time in a soft, feeble voice, "Like this," and he pointed to a dark-brown spot in his hand. "I had several of these, and the doctor said they might be melanoma, so he did a biopsy, but it was not malignant. I have a whole bunch of these, but I guess they're okay."

"Well," I told him, "if they had not been okay, you could have had serious problems. Real melanoma of the skin can be quite bad and can even kill you, so it's good they did the biopsies, but eye melanoma, if it's discovered early enough, may not be as bad as real skin melanoma and can often be treated and cured. In any case, let's get an ultrasound done to see if this thing in your eye really is a melanoma or not."

I called for the technician, who then took the patient for an A-scan. It gave me a chance to speak with the daughter. "Quantitative A-scan is a great test and easy to do, if you have the right technician to do it. It is painless and can immediately tell us what is inside the tumor. Right now, the most important determination is whether this really is a melanoma, some other tumor, or even a metastasis from some cancer elsewhere in his body. The scan can tell us this, so let's see. It will take about twenty to thirty minutes. Meanwhile, if you don't mind, go and sit in the waiting room, and I'll call you when the test is finished."

About forty minutes later, all three of us were back in the exam room. The A-scan had suggested with at least 95 percent accuracy that indeed we were dealing with a melanoma—four millimeters in height and seven millimeters in diameter at its base—a medium-sized malignancy, according to COMS criteria. I started to explain the next steps we should take.

"First of all, you should know that a tumor like this can be treated. There are two types of treatment, one is with radiation and the other is with surgical removal, which really means that the eye has to be removed. At this time, we are involved with a national study to see which treatment works best. So if you want to be in this study, we will decide for you which treatment you get, emphasizing the word *we*. We do this in a random manner, sort of like flipping a coin, because we really do not know which is better, but we do know that treatment is much better than no treatment."

I then spent the next twenty minutes discussing the treatments and the study. It always took considerable time to explain clinical studies to patients. In the case of eye melanoma, there was the additional problem that the two treatments were so different. In one case, the patient would lose an eye, which was a frightening prospect for anyone, especially for the family, which was often afraid of what the patient might look like after the surgery. Reassurance concerning the excellent cosmetic result of this operation was usually required to make that choice palatable. Still, some patients actually preferred eye removal, because it removed the whole cancer right away. Intuitively, patients thought that this would guarantee a cure, even though we told them that microscopic metastases, or spread to other organs, presently undetectable, might have already occurred. Radiation, on the other hand, which also involved surgery, attacked the cancer more slowly. After the implantation of a radioactive plaque next to or behind the eye and the subsequent removal of the plaque seventy to a hundred hours later, the tumor would then shrink over the next few months, turn into a ball of scar tissue, or disappear completely, leaving an internal scar behind. This comparatively minor surgery, which was relatively noninvasive and remarkably easy for patients to undergo, seemed at first to be preferred by most patients and their families. However, the thought that some cancer cells were still viable for a while in the eye with the potential for systemic spread caused some patients to prefer eye removal.

As expected, the patient's daughter wanted to have nothing to do with any study, any experimentation on her father. I again emphasized that neither treatment was an experiment. I told her that, until now, some tumor doctors had always used enucleation and that others usually favored radiation.

"Well, you must know which you prefer," she asserted. "If this was *your* father, which would you do?"

"Frankly, I would put my father in the study" was my reply. "But it's not necessary to decide now. There is plenty of time to make the choice. First, we have to do some preliminaries. We need a good physical exam on your father to make sure he is otherwise okay. Do you have an oncologist, a cancer specialist, that you know in Harlingen? An oncologist is really the best at this time. He would know where to look for metastases. That's important. I want to know that there is no other tumor or cancer anywhere else."

"Yes, we have a very good doctor," she responded. "He has been my dad's doctor for many years."

"Is he a tumor specialist?" I asked.

"No, but he is very good and very thorough. He'll be just fine."

I raised my eyebrows. "I guess that's okay, if you say so." *If she was not a nurse, I would never agree to that,* I thought to myself.

"By the way," I asked the patient, "do you have any other bumps or lumps anywhere other than the pigmented skin spots we talked about? And how about any recent new complaints such as stomach discomfort, breathing problems, or difficulty when you go to the bathroom?"

The daughter immediately spoke, almost interrupting my last sentence.

"We'll let our doctor in Harlingen ask those questions, and as far as any lumps and bumps go, there's just the lipoma on the back of his neck, which he has had for years. Here, Dad, turn your head and show the doctor." The patient turned his head to the right, and I could see a bump on his neck, just above his collar, the size of a large grape. The skin overlying it was normal, and as I could feel, it was soft to the touch, round, and seemingly not connected to the overlying skin. I agreed that it felt like a lipoma, a fatty but benign tumor, not uncommon in the elderly. In fact, it felt identical to the numerous lipomas that our family Vizsla dog had for many years before she died of old age.

"Are you sure this has not grown recently?" I wanted to know. "No, it's the same." The patient nodded in agreement.

"Still," I suggested, "since it would be so easy to do, why don't you arrange for a biopsy? Then we'll be sure. You, as a nurse, must know some surgeon over there in Harlingen who can do that easily in the office."

"We'll see what our doctor says" was the assertive reply.

"Okay, I guess."

After the visit, the patient and his daughter returned home. She arranged for the visit with the general practitioner, who reportedly performed a thorough physical examination. Even if he had never had an eye melanoma patient before, I assumed that all the appropriate history, physical examination, and blood tests were done to rule out metastases or other cancers. I also knew that he would observe the pigmented skin lesions and the neck tumor, which he felt were all benign.

Meanwhile, during the ten days it took for all the tests to be done, I hoped that a decision would be made about the study or whether enucleation or radiation would be chosen. On day 6, I called the daughter to make certain that she had managed to get the doctor's appointment and also to emphasize again that being in the COMS study might be the optimal choice. The study would then decide which treatment would be given. "We know that both treatments worked a lot of the time with medium-sized melanomas, and neither treatment was experimental. We just did not know if one treatment was a little better than the other.

"Therefore, since there is no scientific basis for choosing one therapy over the other, you can avoid the possibility that you will make the wrong choice—a thought that you may not want to live with for the rest of your life. For example, let's assume that you choose radiation and that your father dies of metastatic cancer a few years later. You will not be able to avoid thinking that you should have chosen enucleation. You might blame yourself. However, if you let the study, the flip of the coin, decide—let luck or God decide—you will be blameless. Thinking like that has given several of my patients, especially church-going patients, great comfort. And by the way, don't you think it would be wise to get that neck biopsy done, even though we all think that it will be negative?"

On the tenth day following the initial visit, I saw the patient and daughter again.

"Our doctor cleared Dad," she said. "There is nothing wrong with him. Here is the report." She briskly produced a paper from her handbag, like a magician pulling a rabbit out of a hat.

The report was a summary of the findings: normal blood count, borderline normal liver function tests, normal PSA (test for prostate cancer) for his age, and normal chest x-ray.

The physical exam mentioned the skin lesions and the neck lipoma; clear lungs; an easily palpable, possibly enlarged liver, compatible with the patient's long history of high alcohol intake; and an otherwise negative abdominal and rectal exam. Peripheral pulses were slightly irregular, but his heart sounds were normal, as was the blood pressure. The summary stated, "All tests normal or acceptable, no evidence of other cancers or metastases. No special surgical risk." It was signed by Thomas Beauregard, MD, family practitioner. There was no mention of any neck biopsy or of an abdominal scan, both of which had been discussed but felt to be unnecessary, according to the daughter. The report clearly had been written for a layperson, the type of summary that doctors these days hand to patients at the end of a visit, not the kind of communication that physicians have with one another. Especially the sentence "all tests were normal or acceptable" would have been unheard of in a professional discussion. There were no details or numbers.

What in the world does acceptable *mean?* I thought. *Acceptable to whom?* "Should I call Dr. Beauregard for more details?" I asked.

"Oh, I don't think so. He and I went through all the numbers, and they were fine."

I should probably trust her report, given that she is a nurse, I thought to myself, with some unease.

"And we have chosen to have the eye removed. At first Dad didn't want that, wanted nothing to do with that, but then I convinced him. I told him—just like you had said, Doctor—that it was not a big operation and that it would not be painful and that with the prosthetic eye in place, he would look very normal. But at least then we know that the tumor is gone and can't do any more harm. He can then live his natural life out without worry. He may still live a long time." She patted her father on the knee. "Dad is in very good health, you know. He is small, not overweight, has never had any heart problems." Another pat on the knee. "Dad, you might live to be a hundred—another twenty-seven years!"

The enucleation was scheduled for the following week and went smoothly. I had already called Dr. Adelsohn, the referring ophthalmologist, to ask when he wanted to do the operation himself, since it required no special equipment and was well within the expertise of any ophthalmic surgeon, but he told me to go ahead and do it. "I have not done an enucleation for years. I like doing cataracts. Much better for the soul."

After surgery, the pathology report confirmed the tumor to be a mixed cell melanoma of the choroid, which I reported to the daughter. Six weeks later, the wound had healed, and the patient was fitted with a prosthesis, painted to match his other eye. He seemed very pleased and confided in me that he was glad to have chosen enucleation. "It wasn't really bad at all."

Because Harlingen was many hours from our office in San Antonio, I arranged for follow-up appointments with Dr. Adelsohn's office and also spoke to him on the telephone. I suggested that he see the patient in about three months and told him that, at the time of surgery, no extraocular extension of the tumor had been noted, so I did not expect a local recurrence in the orbit. I also mentioned the assertive personality of the daughter and suggested that he insist that she take her father for a medical checkup every six months, no matter what she thought.

"That's what I told her, and I'd love it if you told her the same. Thanks so much for helping me with the follow-up on this patient.

With the daughter's job as a nurse supervisor, she really can't take the time to bring her father all the way to San Antonio."

About three months later, I called Dr. Adelsohn again to get a report of the patient's progress. Apparently, the appointment had been cancelled because of illness. I decided to call the daughter, whom I finally spoke to, after leaving several messages.

"Dad has been very sick. Some GI problem. He can't keep anything down, has no appetite, and has lost weight. You know how small he is already. He is very weak. I'm taking him to another doctor in Galveston tomorrow."

"Let me know what happens," I insisted.

About ten days later, she called back. She was upset.

"How can this happen? Dad is full of cancer. They say it's metastatic melanoma. They biopsied everything—his liver, his abdomen, even the lipoma on his neck. It's all cancer. Why didn't you insist that we do those biopsies before? You could have arranged it so easily in San Antonio. Then we would have known earlier and maybe treated him with chemo or something and saved his life or even avoided having to put him through that miserable eye operation. How would you like to spend the last three months of your life with only one eye? Now he's got acute liver failure. They've given him less than a month to live. Thank God they've got him sedated."

"I am so sorry to hear that. I guess he already had cancer spread when we operated. Not that we knew that. In retrospect, it would have been nice to know that, but we didn't. Remember we talked about a biopsy . . . Well, we never did it."

"You should have insisted."

The phone call ended abruptly after that comment. I sat back on my chair, staring at nothing. Yes, I had mismanaged this patient. I had deviated from the rigorous protocol that I always followed, which included consulting with an oncologist and scheduling that neck biopsy myself before undertaking any treatment. The oncologist and I would certainly have ordered a liver biopsy or liver scan, since the patient did have an enlarged liver. Then I should have had the biopsies interpreted by a reliable pathologist familiar with metastatic melanoma. I should never have permitted myself to be intimidated by the nurse's strong opinions and never used the distance to Harlingen as a reason. I might have saved the patient an operation, even though I might not have saved his life.

Mea culpa. Mea maxima culpa.

Chapter 5

BLACK SPOTS

I finally found a painter who was cheap and had a pretty good reputation in the valley. He was in his early thirties, a small thin man with a beaked nose yet small face and chin, who smiled easily and spoke simply. He was the only son of a neighboring farmer down the road, where he lived in small, one-room camp, as he called it, on his parents' property. He helped his father milk the sixteen cows and manage the small twenty-acre farm, which was largely made up of six small meadows cut into the hilly woodland. I don't know how much schooling he had had, but I doubt that he ever graduated from high school. That, together with his short stature and peculiar bird-like face, probably precluded a full adult life with wife and children. His high voice was also unusual, as if he had never been through puberty.

To earn enough money to support himself, he became a house painter. Most of his work was done in the valley, where everyone seemed to know him. He was someone I needed. I had just bought, even though I was still an eye resident, a small ski cabin near Hell's Creek ski area in Vermont. After gutting the place and redoing the inside walls with sheetrock, with which my resident friends helped me on the weekends, I needed a painter who was cheap and could do his work while I was at the hospital.

Wilbur did a good job, and every weekend, I would see the slow progress he was making. Then one Saturday morning, I noticed that he must have spilled a can of paint on the floor near the kitchen. I asked him about it when he came over for his weekly inspection. He was very apologetic, but I assured him that it didn't matter, because the floor was still unfinished plywood. A few weeks later, as Wilbur was painting the newly hung door to the bedroom, where a new wall-to-wall carpet had just been installed, he knocked over a small ladder, on which his paint can was standing. I heard the noise and ran upstairs to see what happened. He was sitting on his knees with an old towel, trying to mop up the paint from the rug. When he looked up, he seemed to be crying.

During the following two weeks, the paint spills made me wonder what was wrong with Wilbur. It seemed so unlikely that a professional painter would spill paint regularly, if ever.

When I saw him the following weekend, I spoke to him, "Don't worry about those paint spills. They don't matter, and we got all the paint off the rug, didn't we?"

He nodded. "Yes, I know, but still . . ."

"I'm just wondering if you feel okay. Are your hands steady? Do me a quick favor, just stretch out your hands for a second."

He obliged.

"Well, that's certainly not the problem. How is your eyesight?"

"Very good, I think. I can read all the small print on the paint cans just fine, and you know I drive a car and have had no accidents."

"Well, that's good. Let me check one other thing. Do you mind?"

"What?"

I was now standing in front of him, face-to-face. With my left index finger on the end of my nose, I said, "Look here at the tip of my nose."

He did so with both eyes open. With my other hand held way to one side and my fingers wiggling, I asked him to tell me when he saw those fingers. I then moved my right hand closer to my left. "Tell me as soon as you see my fingers wiggling. How about now?"

THE EYE: WINDOW TO BODY AND SOUL

There was no response until my right hand was nearly touching my left. *My god,* I thought. *He has no peripheral vision.*

What I had just done was a very crude visual field test, and it showed a gross bilateral peripheral visual field defect. I repeated the test with one eye at a time and was able to reconfirm my finding. Now I knew why he had knocked over the paint cans. He couldn't see anything to either side!

"You have a little trouble seeing to the side, don't you?"

"I guess so, but it doesn't really bother me."

"Next weekend, Wilbur, I'll bring a little gadget with me so I can check one other thing. You know I'm studying to be an eye doctor, so this is good practice for me. You're helping me out." We both laughed, as the attention shifted from him to me.

The following weekend, I brought dilating eye drops to facilitate my retinal examination with an indirect ophthalmoscope. Now, it became clear where the problem was. The abnormality was in the retina of both eyes. There was diffused above-normal pigmentation in all areas of the retina, especially in the periphery. The pigment was prominent along the retinal blood vessels, which were abnormally narrowed. The optic nerve looked white instead of pink, indicating atrophy. The diagnosis was obvious. This was very likely retinitis pigmentosa, an irreversible and untreatable condition. The fact that it was so advanced at such an early age probably meant that it was genetically autosomal recessive. This would mean that Wilbur would have had to get the gene from both his parents. I thought about the likelihood of such an occurrence. Wilbur's family on both his parents' side was from the Hell's Creek Valley. His mother had been one of sixteen children, but his father only had one sibling, a sister. However, all four grandparents were from very large valley families with more than six children each, and many of them married in their teens. Frequently, the oldest child in a family had a child of his/her own that was the same age as the child's youngest brother or sister. For several generations since the early 1800s, almost no one had moved from the valley. They were all mostly farmers or construction workers who were undereducated but employed, content to stay in their beautiful environment. I could easily imagine that some inbreeding might have occurred in such an isolated social island. That might have brought out recessively transmitted medical conditions, such as this early onset retinitis degeneration which would, in a more mobile society, be very rare.

To make sure that my diagnosis was correct and no treatment was available, I arranged for a neighbor to drive Wilbur to Boston, where the Massachusetts Eye and Ear Infirmary (MEEI) had special expertise in this diagnosis. The confirmation came quickly in a phone call from a friend working in the retinitis pigmentosa lab at the MEEI.

During the next several years, Wilbur's central vision also began to decrease, as was expected. He stopped painting but continued to help at the farm. By the time he was forty-two, he was almost totally blind with some light perception and motion vision. Even then, with help of a cane, which he learned to use by himself, he got around the barn and continued to milk the cows twice a day. Sometimes, one could see him walk the last cow into the barn at milking time, leading him as he held on to its tail. His countenance never changed, he still had that childlike easy smile.

In his late forties, he had an accident and fell against the metal side of a hay bailer, which had been parked in an unusual place. He hurt his head severely and became unconscious. I heard later that he never recovered.

The retinal pigmentation Wilbur had was quite typical of RP, but pigmentation (black spots) in the retina varies a lot in appearance and occurs in many disparate conditions.

Black or dark-brown spots usually originate in the retinal pigment epithelium (RPE), a single cell layer under the retina. Among other functions, the RPE acts like a garbage collector, mopping up the metabolic excrement of the busy, metabolically active retina.

In a normal fundus (back of the eye), with the RPE being undisturbed, the pigment is diffused, like the dark filter of sunglasses. However, when the RPE is disturbed, the pigment stops being evenly distributed and instead clumps in certain places and disappears in others, giving the fundus a mottled look. In some conditions, the RPE cells can even proliferate and form very dark clumps or even small black or brown tumors.

Because the RPE is very sensitive, there are many ocular conditions which can disturb it, many of which are totally benign and stable and do not interfere with vision. If unilateral, they tend to be due to local monocular events, such as an injury or an infection. Binocular pigment disorders are more likely due to systemic conditions, even as benign as simple aging. They could also be due, as was the case with Wilbur, to a genetic disorder such as retinitis pigmentosa.

I remember one patient who had unusual pigmentation in the fundus, which did not affect vision but was a signal of a systemic disorder elsewhere in the body. There were small clumps of pigment, which looked like the footprint of an animal in mud. Some observers have called them bear tracks, and that denotation has stuck. I saw these during a routine examination of a fifty-seven-year-old attorney, whom I had never met before. Joel Taylor was getting a yearly eye checkup, having been told that he was now at an age when he should see an ophthalmologist and not an optometrist. He was no longer seeing eye doctors for optical problems such as reading or computer glasses or contact lenses. He was now at the age for cataracts, glaucoma, vitreous and retinal detachments, eye tumors, and macular degeneration. His family doctor had told him that he should start getting used to seeing an ophthalmologist yearly.

Because it was his first visit, I dilated his pupils and performed a complete eye examination. That's when I saw the bear tracks, which were obvious in one eye but less apparent and very peripheral in the second eye. The bilaterality was important because it indicated the potential for a systemic association with a condition of the colon, so-called familial polyposis or Gardner's syndrome. Such patients develop multiple polyps of the colon, known precursors of colon cancer.

After the otherwise normal exam, Joel and I had a discussion, which unfortunately was brief. He told me that his grandfather may have died of colon cancer, but he was very old, "well over eighty-five."

He followed that up with "If you get to be that old, you've got to die of something."

"Have you ever had a colonoscopy?"

"No, but I don't really want one. My brother just hated his, and it hurt! Of course, it was negative, a total waste of time. And then, didn't you hear about the television anchor who died from a colonoscopy? They perforated his gut! That should have been quite a lawsuit!"

Joel was obviously irritated, and he quickly terminated the conversation. "Sorry, Doc, I gotta go. I have a hearing in about fifteen minutes."

After he left, I wondered how I could get his attention and convince him to do the right thing: get his colon examined.

The next day, my receptionist informed me that Joel's family doctor was internist Max Packer, a good friend of mine. I called Max, and he agreed to telephone Joel about the colonoscopy. Later, Max called me back at home to tell me that the test had been ordered and scheduled.

A few days before the test, I got another call from Max, who had been contacted by Joel, who was complaining about the gallon of fluid he had to drink the night before. He also didn't like the fact that he couldn't eat breakfast or even have coffee. He apparently had an important meeting in that afternoon of March 12 and was concerned that he might not be in top form. "Is this really necessary? Can't you tell in some simpler way if I have polyps?" Max had again convinced Joel to go through with it but wasn't sure that his convincing would last more than a few hours. That last comment made me put Joel's home phone number in my calendar, for the day before the test.

When that day arrived, after I came home from the office and was having my routine 6:00 PM glass of Pinot Gris, I telephoned Joel at his home. His wife answered and told me that he hadn't started drinking that gallon of lemon water yet.

"I just made a quick little supper for us both just in case he doesn't drink the stuff."

"Mrs. Taylor, please don't give him the chance to back out. He is a stubborn guy, does not like to be told what to do, and doesn't like doctors much. He certainly doesn't like medical procedures, but this one is quite benign and very important. I want you to help me help him! Please, please, please!"

"Do you want to talk to him yourself?"

"No, that's not necessary, if you promise that you'll do your job. You can always tell him that I called."

"I'll take care of it," she affirmed.

"Good Luck."

She chuckled.

About ten days later, I got copies of the colonoscopy results. Many polyps were found in the descending colon and multiple biopsies were done while some of the smaller lesions were cauterized. Two of the biopsies were positive for colon cancer. I called Max Packer, who had already referred the patient to an oncologist.

The patient was now in the hands of the University Cancer Center, which orchestrated a battery of local and systemic treatments. Two years later, the oncologist declared Joel Taylor cancer free, although he would continue to be checked with multiple colonoscopies for the rest of his life.

About four years after my initial encounter, I noted the name Joel Taylor on my patient list. I saw him promptly and asked how everything was.

"Great, except that my vision, especially at night, is a little blurry." Since he offered no other history, I went through the eye exam methodically. Other than the bear tracks, which were still there, everything was normal except for early signs of cataract in both eyes. His vision, however, was still 20/20 in each eye. We discussed cataract and its slow inevitable progression and that, if he lived long enough, he might need surgery. As he got up to leave, I could not resist asking, "What finally happened with that colon cancer you had?"

He turned around quickly to face me. "You know, I could never believe that you saw something in my eyes that forced me to go through all those miserable tests. It's a good thing that you were even more stubborn than I was. So now I am fine . . . in great shape." Then he smiled and put his hand on my shoulder.

"Thanks, Doc, you were right."

Part IV

LISTEN AND YOU WILL SEE

Chapter 1: New Knowledge 107
Chapter 2: Insult.. 114
Chapter 3: Playing God 120
Chapter 4: Chief Complaint 126
Chapter 5: The Patient Knows Best 133

Chapter 1

NEW KNOWLEDGE

On December 27, a day when we always left a few appointment slots open on my schedule to accommodate patients who needed to be seen urgently following the holidays, I saw Sean O'Leary again, just as I had the previous year. I remembered the Irishman's name and his unusual story about seeing a black spot, which interfered with his reading while at church on Christmas Day. At that time, he had a small retinal hemorrhage close to the central macula of one eye, which fortunately cleared up during the subsequent six weeks. I never really understood why this had happened, but he and I agreed that hard rubbing of his eye, when he cried as he became emotional during the musical Christmas service, could have been the cause, especially in someone with the vascular fragility of a diabetic, which he was.

"Hello again, Doctor, and Merry Christmas. I'm back again with the same problem." He spoke with the brogue accent, rolling his r's and almost singing his vowels.

"Nice to see you again. I remember you from last year. Were you able to contain your emotions in church this time?" I smiled.

"Not really. I suppose that I'll go a bit blind every Christmas. You know, last year wasn't even the first time I had this. I had it a wee bit two years ago and perhaps also four years ago. I wager that

I am your only patient with Christmas blindness. It reminds me of an acquaintance in Cork who, every Easter, gets an itchy roughness in the palms of his hands, which bleeds for a bit for a few days when he scratches it and then goes away. I suppose we are both religious freaks! What do you say?"

"I don't know, but that's really interesting. What does your priest think? Have you told him about it? "What else do you do at Christmastime that you don't do the rest of the year?"

"Well, of course, we get together with the family and both kids and now our two grandchildren, who are twelve and fourteen, to exchange presents and have dinner, after which we go to midnight Mass, which starts at 11:00 PM and is a great musical event. I even participate in the service and play a trumpet voluntary at the beginning of Mass. It's the only time I still play the trumpet. As a young bloke, I played a lot, even in the school band, but no more."

"So that's probably the reason for your eye bleeding." I spoke slowly and thoughtfully.

"When you blow the trumpet, especially on a long and sustained note, you are really straining, blowing against a barrier or resistance, and raising the vascular pressure in the veins of your head incredibly. You know that when you blow the trumpet, especially if you don't do it all the time, your face may get flushed and the veins on your forehead or temple or neck may really become distended or prominent. In medicine, we call this the Valsalva maneuver, where the pressure within the veins in your head, including your eyes, becomes very high. With you and your diabetes, these blood vessels are especially fragile and may leak some blood, which is probably what happens every Christmas. You have been fortunate so far that the bleeding has been so slight and that it has cleared up by itself."

He looked at me intently, seeming to understand. "So should I give up the trumpet?"

"Well, sure, I would recommend it. Why don't you pay for your grandson to get trumpet lessons? Then he can play in church, and you can all go listen to him. Just don't be his teacher!"

He laughed. "I'll think about it."

A few weeks later, when the blood had cleared, I ordered a fluorescein angiogram, which demonstrated several possible source points for bleeding in both retinas. Using the argon laser, I treated these sources and continued to warn the patient against further trumpet playing.

Two years later, after missing a couple of appointments, he again returned with the same Christmas symptoms, this time with a massive hemorrhage in one eye. Vitrectomy surgery, which was then a newly developed surgical procedure, was able to remove the blood and give him 20/20 vision again. He was lucky, but he still had not given up the trumpet. He proudly informed me, however, that his grandson was taking trumpet lessons.

The following year, Sean and his grandson, now seventeen years old, performed the trumpet voluntary together as a duet. He was very proud and wanted to share his pleasure with me on the telephone. "And I had no bleeding in my eyes," he asserted. "Perhaps I didn't have to blow so hard because there were two of us."

"Thanks for calling me, but I still think that it's not a good idea to keep doing this. This year, you were just lucky. Promise me that next year, you'll let your grandson do it by himself."

"We'll see" was the prophetic response.

Sean's story turned out not to be the only such experience I had with diabetic patients not heeding my warning about ocular hemorrhages, which could always, even with laser treatments or invasive vitrectomy surgery, lead to permanent blindness.

In the late seventies, I recall having a twenty-nine-year-old female patient who was a physical therapist, with whom I felt an immediate kinship. After all, she was a member of the medical profession, and her direct no-nonsense conversational manner, coupled with a perpetual smile, was disarming. This was a girl you could talk to, and she would understand.

She had been referred because of her diabetic eye problems, which had already needed multiple laser treatments to control bleeding from the retina. She had recently moved to Texas and needed retinal follow-up care. She had juvenile diabetes since age six and, by the time she graduated from high school, was noted to have recurrent vitreous cavity hemorrhages. The fluorescein angiography had shown large areas in the retina of capillary dropout (small blood vessel closure), typical of poorly controlled diabetes. Also typical was the growth of new blood vessels (neovascularization) at the edge of these avascular areas, an attempt of the body to repair the damage. However, in the retina, this type of repair doesn't really work, since the neovascularization grows on the surface of the retina instead of inside the retina and thus does little to nurture the oxygen-deprived retina itself. It is this neovascularization that is fragile and easily bleeds, especially when stressed. The treatment at that time was to destroy it with laser, and Sylvia had already been extensively treated in both eyes.

As I walked from the waiting room, where I picked her up, to the exam room, I noticed how athletic she seemed to be, with broad shoulders and small hips, walking quickly with long strides, very tall and erect, almost masculine. She got to room 3 before me.

"Is this where I go?" She was impatient. "Yes, go ahead and sit on the big chair."

As she sat down, she reached to shake my hand.

"I'm Sylvia Henderson, but please call me Butch. That's what my father called me as a baby. I guess he really wanted a boy. Now, everyone calls me that." Her handshake was firm.

"I guess you know why I'm here. Dr. Gomez must have told you. I had another vitreous hemorrhage last week when I was moving from Albuquerque. It's my right eye this time. I thought we might be finished with all this stuff by now, but maybe it was the stress of moving that did it."

She continued to speak as I examined her. Both eyes had hundreds of retinal laser scars, and there was some blood on the retinal surface in the right eye near the central macula, which explained her symptoms.

"Well, Butch, I think that this small bleed will absorb, and then, in a few weeks, we will repeat the angiography to find the leak, and maybe do some more laser. But tell me, did you move all your stuff yourself or did you get a mover?"

THE EYE: WINDOW TO BODY AND SOUL

"Are you kidding?" she quickly retorted. "I can't afford a mover, and right now, I just started a new job, which is only part-time. I haven't even gotten paid yet. I work for the Santa Anna Clinic. Hopefully, I can have the same arrangement as I did in New Mexico—work part-time as a physical therapist and be a personal trainer in a gym the rest of the time. That makes pretty good money, and at the same time, I can use the gym for myself. I just love to exercise. My body needs it. I go crazy if I miss even a day, and I'd get fat also." She smiled even more.

"So you carried a lot of heavy boxes and stuff when you moved?"

"Well, yes, but it wasn't too bad. Nothing over fifty pounds anyway."

Her response gave me a chance to pontificate on the hazards of straining versus training. Remembering the experience with my trumpet-playing patient, I told her that whenever she lifted anything, especially if she stooped down to lift something heavy, she would increase the venous pressure in her head and risk a bleed.

"I know, I know," she responded impatiently.

"And many people, when they do lifting, hold their breath, a typical Valsalva maneuver, which makes it worse."

"But, Doctor, I am an athlete, and I teach athletics. I know all that, and I try never to hold my breath, so I don't strain. Even when I lift weights, I keep breathing normally."

Following that visit, I saw her again six weeks later, performed some laser treatment, and reiterated my advice, "Just be careful. Remember that just lying down flat increases the venous pressure in your head, including your eyes, and that straining, holding your breath while lifting weights, makes that worse. You should probably never do bench presses and instead stand up if you are doing weights. Can you do that? You know you have been lucky so far, but a major bleed might not clear up so easily by itself and could even blind you if the surgery you might need to clear it up isn't successful. I've seen it happen in other patients, and I don't want it to happen in you."

"OK, OK, Doctor. I hear you." She was still smiling as she quickly got out of the chair and bounced jauntily toward the waiting room and exit.

Three months later, she cancelled her appointment, giving the receptionist the message for me that she was doing fine. Then, a couple of months later, she called, very upset, and needed to be seen right away because she had gone blind suddenly, as she told the desk clerk on the phone.

I saw her later that day, adding her to the afternoon schedule. A girlfriend, who was holding her by the hand and carefully steering her toward a waiting room chair, accompanied her. It was obvious that she couldn't see much out of either eye.

The exam on that day was brief and simply showed massive bleeding in both eyes. The blood was a very dark red-brown and probably clotted. It seemed unlikely that these hemorrhages would clear by themselves. The decision was thus made to do vitrectomy surgery, one eye at a time, over the next couple of weeks, to remove the blood and the vitreous gel from the eyes and then perform more laser if vascular leaks could be found.

During this time, I had the chance to question Butch about what she had done to cause the bleeding.

"I was just lifting weights, that's all. You had told me not to lie down and not to hold my breath. And so I was standing up and doing arm curls and also lifting the weights over my head. You know that I have to exercise. Uh, uh, that's just me. I go crazy if I don't, but I was being a good girl."

"Well, maybe weightlifting is not the right thing for you. I'm sure you can find other kinds of exercise to do."

That week, the surgery, although invasive, went surprisingly well in both eyes, leaving a few stray red blood cells behind, which cleared up during the subsequent weeks. Some additional laser was done, and her vision returned to 20/20. She was exuberant with the result, as was I, and seemed to have learned the lesson that straining was to be avoided.

She modified her exercise routine and remained bleed-free for the next fifteen years, when she moved to another city and I lost track of her. However, about three years after her surgery, some publications began to appear in the ophthalmic research literature, which clearly demonstrated that the blood pressure in athletes during weightlifting can rise dramatically, even fourfold, to levels which can cause, although rarely, brain or retinal hemorrhages, even in normal people without fragile vessels. Although the mechanism of this sudden and extreme high blood pressure was not clearly understood, the fact that it happened was incontrovertible. It made me think that I should tell Butch, whom I had not forgotten, about this research.

Fortunately, my secretary was able to locate her. I called her and was able to share the new knowledge with her. She was surprised and grateful for my call and pleased to have found an explanation for her ocular hemorrhages.

"Too bad I didn't know this earlier. I would've warned you not ever to do any weightlifting at all. Instead, I told you not to lie flat or with your head down and not hold your breath. Now we know that weightlifting can make blood pressure go sky high and should definitely be avoided by people like you!"

Chapter 2

Insult

"Do I really need to answer all these questions about my diabetes? I'm just here for an eye exam. You sound like my regular doctor."

It was not an unusual comment from a patient, especially one who tended to be noncompliant and didn't want to be reminded of that. In this case, the noncompliance was obvious. The patient was obese and clearly out of shape, having trouble walking and getting into the exam chair. He carried a plastic grocery bag, which he hung on the arm of the chair, and I could just imagine the food he was carrying around in it so that he could snack anytime. It was always the fat people who brought food, often candy or cookies, giving the excuse that they needed sweets to prevent a hypoglycemic attack. His dislike of my questions irritated me, but I persisted and told him that eye doctors and internists or diabetologists always work together, because good blood sugar control in an adult-onset diabetic could often diminish all the vascular complications of diabetes, which cause kidney failure, amputation, and especially blindness.

"Since you want me to be your eye doctor, you have got to understand that it is my job to prevent you from going blind, and the best way for me to do that is to prevent you from getting the blood vessel problems to begin with, rather than treat the vascular bleeding problems after they have already occurred. You must know that diabetes is the most common cause of blindness in America! So let's prevent it, because after you start bleeding in your eyes, it may be too late because the treatment may not always work."

The patient grunted disapprovingly.

"So tell me the name of your diabetic doctor so that I can be in touch with him."

"It's Dr. Jorge Gonzalez. He's in this same building, the Texas Diabetes Institute, downstairs on the first floor."

"Well, that's good. That makes it easy. He and I share a lot of patients."

"Yes, do talk to him, and you may find out some surprising things about me." His words were spoken aggressively.

"Is it about your weight and your diet? You know that I have several patients who lost weight, started to exercise, and got in really good shape and then even stopped having diabetes. They never developed the eye problems. In one patient who did have some diabetic signs in the retina, the eye problems resolved completely once he got control over his life. It was amazing and wonderful, and I never had to treat any diabetic eye retinopathy in him. Never had to use lasers or anything."

"You're goddam right that it's about weight. Why don't you stop your preaching and look at this?"

He took the grocery bag off the arm of the chair and pulled an old newspaper out of it.

"Read it. It's from several months ago, and you'll see that I know more about losing weight and getting better diabetic control than you do. So instead of talking down to me and insulting me, read the article. It's not long." He pushed it into my hand.

The paper showed a photo of an extremely obese person being lifted by some sort of mechanical sling out of a bed. The article indicated that the patient weighed close to eight hundred pounds and was totally incapacitated, unable to walk or even move much and had to be lifted by what looked like a crane in order to defecate or urinate.

He had an oxygen tube in his nose and could barely lift his arms to bring food to his mouth.

"Who is this?" I asked.

"That is me about a year ago. That's when I realized that I was going to die before turning forty. Now, I have lost over four hundred pounds, so don't tell me how to lose weight."

"Well, how did you do it? I don't even recognize that you are the same person as the one in the picture."

He abruptly leaned back and pulled his shirt up out of his pants to show me a huge horizontal scar on his abdomen.

"I had several operations. First, they put a band around my stomach, which made me not want to eat very much anymore. After a couple of bites, I felt full. That sure helped. Then, they surgically removed over a hundred pounds of fat from my belly and my upper legs. That left me with a skirt of skin, which hung down almost to my knees. So they removed that a few months later, and it weighed more than a hundred pounds. That made it possible for me to start moving again. So now they have me on an exercise program, which I do every day, except Sundays, for at least four hours. You know that you have this little gym here at the Institute. That's where I do it. I've got nothing else to do. I lost my janitor job years ago, so now I'm on welfare and live nearby with my mother, who enjoys having me around now that I am getting better. You know I've lost over four hundred pounds. Unbelievable! And the doctors have been wonderful, especially Dr. Krespe, the surgeon, who recently admitted to me that he had never operated to remove so much fat and skin in anybody before. The other people at the gym also can't believe how well I am doing. That's why I carry this newspaper around with me—to show them what is possible."

I let him talk since he seemed to enjoy telling his story of success. As he spoke, his whole demeanor improved and became less belligerent.

"You know that I am down to two hundred and sixty pounds now, which may be obese to you, but it is a hell of a lot better than eight hundred. And I am still losing weight—two pounds a week. I weigh myself every morning before I put any clothes on, and if I haven't lost the two pounds by Sunday morning, I know that I have to lose them that day. That's sometimes tough because not eating at all really screws up your diabetes and can give you an insulin reaction. I take insulin twice a day, and on those Sundays that I can't eat much, I cut down on the dose a little. It seems to work."

"At least on those Sundays you can go to church and pray that it will," I piped up. "Let me take a look at your eyes."

The exam was quick as I zeroed in on the retina, where I would get the most information about his diabetes. To my surprise, the diabetic vascular changes were minimal, consisting only of a few minute hemorrhages and a few microaneurysms, small outpouching on retinal vessels, indicating some vessel wall weakness.

"You're lucky so far," I summarized. "So maybe the timing of your decision to get control of yourself was just right. Keep it up! I wish you the best with your diet, and I do want to apologize for preaching to you even before I had listened to your story. That was stupid of me and, I must say, unusual for me also."

His nod indicated that he heard me and was not disagreeing.

"But since you are doing so well, I think there is a possibility that the retinal hemorrhages may clear up completely. I'd like to be able to tell you so someday, and of course, if they get worse, we can always treat with a laser. So let's stay in touch. I'd like to see you in about three months. How does that sound?"

"That's fine."

I accompanied him to the waiting room, where the receptionist set the appointment date.

During the next few weeks, I thought about my obese patient, knowing that most people on drastic diets are ultimately not successful. At some point, they can't contain their soda, snacks, cookies, and candy craving any more, and they resume their weight-gain pattern. To be and stay successful, some people even need some form of psychotherapy to deal with their depression, which often is the root cause of it all.

When he returned for the next visit, however, my patient was ebullient.

"Before you say anything, Dr. van Heuven, let me tell you that I've lost another twenty-six pounds. I'm now two hundred and thirty-four pounds, and I continue to lose two pounds a week. It's working! My mother thinks that I'm a changed person. She says that I've never been so positive my whole life, even better than I was as a child. Well, I sure feel better than I ever remember feeling. I spend lots of time at the gym. I don't go to the little gym here in this building anymore. I go to the big YMCA gym a few blocks from here, and they gave me a job. They are actually paying me. I take care of the equipment, but half the time, at least four hours a day, I help people use the machines. And then there is one yoga class that I teach with another guy. We always start with a few minutes of meditation. You know meditation is really great." He chuckled.

He also made me smile as I started the exam. Nothing had changed. His retinopathy had not improved, but it was no worse.

During the next year, I kept in touch with him, seeing him every three months, during which he reached his goal of 180 pounds. He told me about a pictorial history of himself, which he had framed and which showed a series of photographs of himself during his remarkable weight loss period. It was proudly displayed behind the sign-in desk of the YMCA.

"It's a great incentive for other people," he assured me.

"I can just imagine," I agreed, and then I started the exam. By now, it had been more than a year since I first saw him, and his retinopathy had almost completely cleared up.

"Your eyes are better, I'm happy to tell you. How's your diabetes?"

"They've taken me off insulin shots and are giving me a pill now. My hemoglobin A1c is normal now, so I'm in pretty good control."

"Congratulations, my friend," I said, and I patted him over the shoulder.

"Now, all I have to do is ask Dr. Krespe to remove this turkey wattle, this loose skin under my chin, and I'll be all set. It will be the new me!"

After this visit, I continued to see this patient for more than six years. By then, he was no longer a diabetic, and all he needed from me was a periodic change of reading glasses.

Chapter 3

Playing God

Lions Clubs in America have always been interested in vision. This highly hierarchical organization is mostly made up of middle-class nonprofessionals who simply like to work together for a common good, and they are highly effective in accomplishing whatever they set out to do and have fun while doing it. Many clubs collect old eyeglass frames, which are then provided to the poor, sometimes in a third world country, but more frequently here at home. Since glass frames rather than the prescription itself are generally the more expensive part of glasses, this is an important activity and permits literally thousands of Americans to get the glasses they need. I have known several poor elderly couples whose only pair of glasses, which they shared, was provided by Lions. But the Lions do many other good deeds. For years, they had regional networks to provide donor corneas for corneal transplantation. Thus, patients with severe corneal opacification, who were nearly blind from this scarring of the front surface of their eyes, could be helped by having a human cadaver cornea transplanted onto their eye, in place of the scarred one. Some of those patients had scarring from trauma; others from infections such as herpes, syphilis, or more common organisms, which invade the corneas of patients wearing their contact lenses too long. Still others suffered from some degenerative diseases of the cornea or of the body.

The organization of these Lions eye banks was complex and involved hospitals and emergency rooms to identify donors; residency training programs to provide personnel to harvest the corneas under sterile conditions; a transportation system by Lions themselves to bring the corneas to the hospital, where they would be used; and an administration to organize this, including the maintenance of a corneal recipient waiting list. The Lions had even made arrangements with some airlines to transport the boxed, refrigerated donor eyes through their pilots, who became personal carriers of this precious cargo.

With the advent of for-profit tissue banks, however, the need for the Lions services became diminished, and they started to look elsewhere for other meaningful projects. That moment coincided with my arrival at the University of Texas Medical School in San Antonio, where I had been asked to form a new independent Ophthalmology Department, no longer under the departmental rule of General Surgery. This was a great opportunity to create a new academic unit encompassing teaching, research, and clinical practice in equally balanced proportions. At that time, the leadership of the Lions of South Texas included several forward-looking individuals, who were leaders in their own communities, who could easily understand the promise of an academic think tank in the field of vision and ophthalmology, which they had already supported in the past. There was one Lion, Lytle Blankenship, a professor, who was particularly attracted to the research part of the academic tripod and was able, over a period of several years, to convince the Lions Clubs to develop a massive fundraising capacity to support basic research, as well as other more easily understood activities, such as a mobile eye-disease screening bus and a low vision clinic.

One of the local Lions, the president of his club, who had become a good friend and steady supporter, one day showed up in my office as a patient. He had recently seen his eye doctor for a routine check of his vision and prescription, but the ophthalmologist, who had dilated his pupils to permit a complete eye exam, had noticed a freckle in his retina, which concerned him. He thus referred Reggie Lewis for another opinion. Reggie had actually suggested the consultation with a retina specialist and had told his doctor that he was a friend of mine.

"Yeah, that's a good idea. Why don't you go see van Heuven? He might not even charge you," the doctor chuckled. "Let him take a picture of it so we can follow this thing in the future, see if it changes or if it grows.

"When it changes, what does it do?" Reggie had asked.

"Well, rarely, it can turn into a tumor, like cancer—a choroidal melanoma, they call it. You've heard of melanoma of the skin, I suppose. Well, this would be a melanoma of the eye, inside the eye. Not half as bad as a real melanoma of the skin, which can often kill you, but a different kind of melanoma, which can be treated very successfully, if we know about it early. But because you cannot see it from the outside, these things can grow quite large before anyone notices and before you lose your vision, so it is good, at this point, to photograph it and keep track of it."

When Reggie showed up at the office, he was ready for the retinal photo. "I came to have my picture taken," he told me as he walked in with his wife, Barbara, whom I had also met many times before, during Lions Clubs meetings. In fact, she was also quite an outspoken leader and supporter of our department as a Lioness, the newly formed women's counterpart of the Lions Clubs, which traditionally had been solely a men's organization.

After the initial pleasantries and some discussion of the very nice recent social at the city's main club, we talked about Reggie's health, as part of the first examination by any ophthalmologist. She handed me the four-page form, which she had already filled out for him. "Here you go, now you have everything." We went over the list of all medical conditions. Reggie was sixty-seven years old, looking somewhat older, and had a long history of troubles with breathing, being short of breath. He had smoked cigarettes for forty years but had recently quit when his doctor threatened him with the thought that he might have to spend the last ten years of his life carrying around an oxygen tank. He also had some cardiac problems, having had stints placed in his coronary arteries on three different occasions. He had some knee problems, which, according to him, made him sway from one side to the other as he walked. I had noticed that when he came in but thought it was mostly due to his weight of at least three hundred pounds. He was a big man, over six feet in height. I supposed that, with such weight, his knees certainly would get a workout. I asked him about his irregular pulse. It was always easy to obtain that information, sitting opposite of the patient in the exam chair, putting my fingers on his wrist as we talked. He told me that he was diagnosed with atrial fibrillation three years before and was on blood thinners ever since. At that time, he had developed heart failure and was given a diuretic pill. He was also taking other medications: Lipitor for cholesterol, some other pill for his borderline diabetes, and a sleeping pill. Then there was a new pill, something experimental, to help control his restless leg syndrome.

As Reggie related his medical history, he seemed to be in his usual jovial mood. "Do you have to go to medical school to learn to take a picture?" he joked, and as he looked sideways to his wife, he said, "Hey, Barb, we have a camera. Maybe *you* could take the picture. It would be a lot cheaper."

Most of the eye exam was normal. His vision was excellent with glasses, and he only had the slightest amount of cataract, obviously not clinically significant and normal for anyone his age. The retina exam did show the freckle, which I explained was really not in the retina but rather under the retina, in the choroid, the vascular layer underneath. The nevus or freckle was about three millimeters across, round and light brown, easy to see against the reddish background, and slightly elevated. An ultrasound examination confirmed the almost-three-millimeter thickness, and the photograph we took through a green filter delineated the edges of the lesion perfectly.

I explained to Reggie that freckles this size are just on the edge of becoming tumors that we should treat. He interrupted me immediately to say, "Well, we don't need to treat this thing now, do we?" I nodded in agreement, knowing that small melanomas like this one were sometimes just observed. Then, should they show any growth whatsoever, radiation or even surgical removal should be done. However, since Reggie was so opposed to any intervention, I agreed that we could check him again in about three months. I knew that Barbara had sensed my discomfort with this decision, but we all agreed to a three-month follow-up appointment. After all, the tumor was less than half a millimeter longer than any pigmented tumor we would simply observe, and Reggie did not want any surgery.

Four months later, I noticed that Reggie had not kept his appointment. I double-checked the dates, and indeed he was a month overdue. When I phoned, Barbara apologized, but he had been sick and his breathing was now worse. "He just got some new heart medicine this week," she explained. "I'll call you back when he's better. Maybe you can see him then."

Three weeks later, they appeared in the office. I had warned the receptionist that should they call, an appointment should be given as soon as possible. Reggie looked older and pale, but his jovial manner had persisted, although when he talked, his breathing was laborious, and he seemed to have gained weight. He barely fit between the armrests of the exam chair and sat straight up, leaning on his elbows to expand his ribcage.

It was now obvious that the tumor had grown. It was now measured over three millimeters in height. We talked about it, but I found myself understating the problem. Perhaps I had already decided that Reggie would never die from this tumor, because his other health problems were potentially much more threatening. It did make me recall, however, the very elderly lady with a retinal detachment in one eye, whom we decided not to operate because of her frailty. She was too much of a surgical risk. Then blind in one eye, she had returned ten years later, at age ninety-six, with a partial retinal detachment in the other eye. That left us no choice but to operate when she was even frailer than before. It had taught me, so I thought, not to predict longevity in anyone.

I gave Reggie another appointment two months hence and then another one three months later. He continued to be unconcerned about his malignant melanoma and never lost his sense of humor. His restless leg syndrome had become worse, and he doubled his medication. Although never verbalized and only hinted through an occasional glance, Barbara and I never interfered with Reggie's desire to ignore his cancer. A few months later, she called to say that he had died of heart failure, sitting in an armchair and watching a football game on television.

Goodbye, Reggie, my friend. I'll see you in heaven. You were right not to worry about your eye tumor.

Chapter 4

Chief Complaint

The most respected and senior faculty member in the department, occupying the Liesenkranz chair of ophthalmology, was noticing some odd symptoms in his vision, which he did not completely understand. At first, it happened during the weekly grand rounds in the brightly neon-lit auditorium but then recurred as he walked into an equally bright VA hospital corridor. At first, he thought he had double vision, and it made him feel unsteady, so he held onto the railing, which extended the full length of the hallway, but then it seemed more like a shimmering in his vision. Everything looked silvery. When he reached the more dimly lit eye clinic, the symptoms went away. All the while, he felt fine otherwise.

He sat down on one of the exam chairs and took his own vision. It was 20/15 in both eyes, even better than 20/20. He also tested his near vision, which was excellent as well, although he had to search a little to see the small letters with his right eye, but once he saw them, he could read even the smallest ones.

He thought about his own medical history. It was essentially negative except for a broken ankle during skiing in his twenties and a hernia repair in his sixties, probably for straining during his regular YMCA gym visits. Now that he was seventy-four years old, he was really in excellent condition, taking only Colace for constipation and

THE EYE: WINDOW TO BODY AND SOUL

an occasional nasal spray for congestion during oak season, because he had been found to be especially allergic to oaks and cats. Most of his friends and almost all his patients had long lists of medications that they took. Keeping it all straight was always a problem for them and daily medication schedules were complicated, often leading to poor patient compliance. He remembered how often he had lectured his students to keep it simple for patients. Don't prescribe some meds three times a day, some four times a day, and still others every eight hours. No patient would ever keep up with that.

No, he was very lucky now. There had been a short time, during his fifties, that he had taken a few pills. He had, because of his father's history of multiple heart attacks, the fourth of which killed him at age sixty-five, that he was part of a study, a small clinical trial run by the chairman of Cardiology, to learn more about the natural history of patients with a strong genetic propensity to cardiac problems. During his fifties, his blood pressure, probably because that was the most busy and stressful time in his academic career, had risen to around 136/86, which was deemed to be borderline hypertensive but was never treated. His pulse was always slow and regular, no more than sixty beats per minute, which he attributed to his many years of jogging. At that time, for about two years, after the guidelines for treatment had been altered, he took a statin drug to lower his cholesterol of 220, but it gave him such bad leg cramps that he substituted a better diet for the pill, which lowered his cholesterol to about 160 and eventually also brought his weight back down from 220 pounds to 184 pounds, which was what he weighed in college.

As he pondered his own history, he weighed himself (182 pounds) and asked one of the residents at the VA to check his blood pressure (124/60) and eye pressure (seveteen millimeters of mercury)—perfectly normal. He felt his own pulse, which was regular—strong and slow—and listened to his own carotid neck arteries with no indication that the flow was impeded. Thus, ruling out some systemic causes which might have contributed to his peculiar dizziness, he decided to make an appointment with one of his ophthalmology colleagues. This was an unusual move for him, since he really had not had a complete eye exam for at least twenty years, when he needed reading glasses. He had felt that he really had no good reason for one because he was always with residents or fellows, whom he taught by letting them examine his own eyes.

It was easiest for him to see the optometrist first. He was the least busy of all the faculty and saw him the next day. The exam was essentially negative, with good vision and no evidence of any eye disorder. Afterward, he went to the photography section, after dilating his own pupils, and let the photo tech take some pictures of both retinas, concentrating on the optic nerve, the central macula, and the midperipheral retina. A few minutes later, he looked at the prints.

The only abnormality was the appearance of his optic nerve, which was somewhat pale but not typical of anything special. During the next few days, his symptoms recurred a couple of times, which prompted him to discuss his situation with a colleague, the glaucoma specialist in the department. He also showed him the optic nerve photos, which he looked at for several minutes.

"Have you ever had high eye pressure?" was his friend's question.

"No, never, and I have my pressure taken all the time by my students."

"You know, the pictures don't really show typical glaucoma changes of the nerve, but they do show some pallor, some optic atrophy, which can be due to glaucoma in some patients. Why don't you get a visual field test done and show me the results? Or have you already had one of those?"

"No, never."

"Let me know when it's done."

The next day, one of the techs performed the test, the result of which was dramatic. The peripheral visual field was severely compromised in both eyes, especially upper nasally and more pronounced in the right eye, where pretty much all vision above very central vision was entirely gone. He wondered why he hadn't ever noted this, but he realized, as he had taught for so many years, that most people don't use their superior visual field much, especially if you are a tall male. What is more noticeable, when looking straight ahead, is when you cannot see things on the sides or below, so you don't bump into things or see a car coming or trip on the sidewalk.

Although the visual field test result was typical for glaucoma, the appearance of his optic nerves was not and could have many other causes. Moreover, his eye pressures had always been normal. He discussed this with another colleague, a neuro-ophthalmologist, who recommended an MRI of the brain, because some cerebral tumors could mimic a glaucomatous field defect. The MRI was done and was normal.

Thus, it seemed that the glaucoma diagnosis was correct. He thought back to the first year of his residency at Yale, when a visiting professor from NIH, Dr. Elmer Ballantyne, had lectured about low-tension glaucoma, which was then thought to be rare. He had explained that glaucoma, which by definition is optic nerve damage from high pressure in the eye, can also occur in some patients with normal pressures. In those patients, that normal pressure may just be too high for those particular eyes. He explained that the vascular theory of glaucoma causation was probably correct and that eye pressure, which is transmitted to all structures within the eyeball, is a force that limits the ability of blood getting into the eye to feed its vital structures, including the optic nerve. It is the systemic blood pressure, which is greater than the eye pressure, that assures good circulation. In normal eyes, therefore, there is a delicate balance between blood pressure and eye pressure. If the eye pressure is too high, blood cannot adequately supply the eye, and glaucoma ensues. If the blood pressure is too low, the same thing may happen.

As Dr. Liesenkranz pondered Dr. Ballantyne's lesson, he thought about his own blood pressure. It had always been normal and even borderline high during the most stressful period in his own career. Now, however, as he was nearing retirement, his blood pressure was lower, even quite low (106/60) at times. He measured it regularly at the gym. Could it be that it was now too low to feed his optic nerve adequately?

He discussed it with his glaucoma colleague, and the decision was made to treat him with glaucoma eye drops, to lower the normal eye pressure even further. Another glaucoma visit was scheduled three months later.

By the time he returned, his symptoms were still increasing in frequency. It was not so much that things seemed to appear silvery but rather that he really had double vision at times, with one image slightly above another. Every time it happened, he covered one eye with his hand and then the other eye. This was true vertical diplopia. The exam indicated good vision in both eyes although he could only read the chart slowly with his right eye. He seemed to be searching for the letters. The visual field test was interpreted as being worse, especially in the right eye, where the defect had encroached upon the center, so the upper half of whatever he looked at, including some of the letters on the chart, was only partially visible. This explained why his reading with that eye was so slow. One of the techs, an orthoptist, a specialist in measuring crossed or misaligned eyes, noted that he really had a vertical misalignment of his two eyes, not really clinically noticeable but definitely measurable. She explained that his central visual field defect had interfered with his binocular reflex, which is the brain's effort to maintain single vision by keeping the eyes aligned, thus preventing double vision. When one eye cannot see well straight ahead, the brain does not get equal input from both eyes and so makes no effort to keep the eyes straight. She recommended that prisms be incorporated in the glasses prescription and would most likely solve the double-vision problem. Another tech then measured the eye pressures, which were well below normal. Why then was he still losing visual field? Why was his glaucoma not controlled? He was worried.

The next appointment, after getting his new glasses, was two months later. His diplopia was cured, but his vision was now worse in the right eye. The visual field showed that he had lost more of his central field in that eye, but fortunately, both his vision and field were stable in the left. His eye pressures were well within the normal range, 16 mm Hg in both eyes, but they had really never been more than 17 or 18, well below the 20–22 considered as the top of the normal range. Could it be that his blood pressure at night, when it had never been measured, was even lower? He remembered again something he had heard from Elmer Ballantyne more than forty years earlier, that whenever a hypertensive glaucoma patient is starting treatment for his high blood pressure, the ophthalmologist should be told about it. In fact, he emphasized that ophthalmologists should always obtain blood pressure information on every patient. He had even suggested that blood pressure measurement be part of every eye exam, especially in adults over forty, when the incidence of glaucoma begins to rise.

He discussed the exam results and his blood pressure concerns with the glaucoma colleague, who immediately called the cardiology office down the hall to see if they had an extra twenty-four-hour blood pressure monitor, which could be borrowed. The answer was affirmative, and so they strapped the cuff and halter monitor to his arm and chest and read the results the following day. Indeed, at about 2:00 AM, for two hours, the blood pressure had dipped to 92/50, very low for an adult male. This could certainly explain the continued vision loss, the two colleagues agreed. They decided to increase the number and frequency of the glaucoma drops. One drop would be taken every twelve hours, another three times daily, and a third at bedtime.

During the following year, there were four more appointments, each one with the same findings. There was no more worsening of visual acuity or visual field. The eye pressures were now twelve or thirteen. Increasingly, he began to believe that his glaucoma was now finally under control.

He felt great relief and wondered how unique his own case was. Certainly, his symptoms were not typical of those described in textbooks, and his optic nerve appeared just atrophic—again, not typical of glaucoma. As months passed, he also began to think that, possibly, many patients with low-tension glaucoma would never know about their very low blood pressure at night. He had never heard of monitoring glaucoma patients for twenty-four hours straight. In fact, no eye doctor, glaucoma specialist or not, had ever taken his blood pressure. Most ophthalmologists didn't even have blood pressure machines in their offices.

It was another year later that he was invited by an Ivy League medical school to give a talk on whatever subject he desired. It was on the occasion of resident day, a yearly event for alumni. He accepted the invitation eagerly and decided to present his own case without mentioning that he was the patient. The speech went well and included many references to the work of Elmer Ballantyne as well as several other American, Swedish, German, and Austrian researchers, who had all written about the blood pressure–eye pressure relationships. He ended his talk with the recommendation that blood pressure be routinely taken, saying sarcastically that one of the first things in a dentist's office is that a tech takes your blood pressure, so why not an ophthalmologist? That comment was apparently not appreciated by some in the audience, judging from the questions. One questioner even accused him of "wanting to upset the apple cart."

It wasn't until several years later that he heard from his glaucoma colleague that, especially in Europe, blood pressure measurements had become routine and twenty-four-hour blood pressure monitoring of glaucoma patients was becoming more common, now that it had been learned that many low-tension glaucoma patients had nocturnal hypotension. It had now been more than fifty years since Elmer Ballantyne had suggested that hypothesis, long before the equipment for such nighttime monitoring was even available. He wondered why or how the pace of progress could have been so slow. Not all new ideas or treatments had been that slow to be adopted. In the early seventies, when the argon laser became available, it was very quickly accepted, and within a couple of years, most ophthalmologists had such a laser. However, laser therapy was a surgical procedure, and new operative interventions always seemed to gain popularity more rapidly than medical nonsurgical breakthroughs. Was that because medical insurances reimbursed doctors so much more for surgery than for medical treatment? He hoped that was not the case.

Chapter 5

THE PATIENT KNOWS BEST

When the resident, as she walked through the waiting room into the office, realized that the seemingly blind patient and his wife smelled bad and were making other patients uncomfortable, she quickly brought the patient into one of the empty exam rooms so as to contain the odor. The couple could not be over forty-five, and the blind man, wearing urine-stained cargo pants, flip-flops, and a grey hoodie, shuffled along partially behind his wife as he held onto her elbow. She was slovenly dressed in a long brownish skirt and a dirty large sweatshirt, which did not cover her bra straps. She was obviously experienced at leading a blind person, as she carefully guided him into the exam chair.

Nancy, the resident, immediately began taking the medical history and performing the routine eye exam. The visual acuity was poor, with no more than hand motion vision in each eye. The external exam and the cornea were normal. The pupils reacted sluggishly to her penlight, and the eye pressures were low, which made her suspect retinal detachments. She instilled the dilating drops to examine the retinas. While she waited the fifteen minutes for the drops to work, she heard the patient's story.

Joe Chernov was the son of Polish immigrants who had ended up in Galveston, Texas, where his father worked in a nearby oil refinery.

The family was poor, and he was an only child, living in an old trailer on the city outskirts. After he started school, his mother got part-time work as a cleaning lady until he was in high school, when she was killed by a pick-up truck as she waited for a bus to take her into town. His father took it hard and started to drink and became abusive. Joe managed to finish high school but then had to get away from his father. He hitchhiked to San Antonio, Texas, where, after being homeless for a few months, he found work as a night watchman at a motel, owned by another Polish immigrant, who felt sorry for him. He didn't get paid much but was able to stay in one of the motel rooms.

"And then life got better," he said as he turned toward his wife. "That's when I met Missy, who was a hotel maid, and we have been together ever since. More than ten years now."

"But what happened to your eyes?" Nancy asked.

"I started to get these flashes of light on my right side, especially in the evening, and then I saw all these floating spots, hundreds of them, and then it was as if a curtain came across my vision in the right eye. But I could still see out of the left one, so I did nothing about it. I couldn't afford a doctor anyway, and it didn't hurt. I thought that it would probably clear up!"

"Missy, didn't you tell him to go to an emergency room or at least see somebody?"

She answered, "He never made much of a deal about it. I guess I, too, thought it would get better again."

Joe continued to talk, "And then two years later, the same thing happened to my other eye, only slightly differently. I saw the flashes, then the floating spots, but the curtain across my left eye came down from above, instead of from below, but then it stopped changing. I would still see and even read and, of course, still work. But then, gradually, the curtain came almost all the way down. It took several months, but then suddenly, I really could not see much anymore. I had to quit my job, but we continued living at the motel, because she was still a maid there. So she took over and has helped and guided me ever since. She's just wonderful, and I would not know what to do without her."

He stopped for a few seconds, as if he needed to think about what he was going to say next. Then he continued.

"As I think about it now, it's funny that my loss of vision almost drew us closer to each other. She even started bringing up the subject of finally getting married, after all these years. Why in the world would anyone want to marry a blind man? I kept saying."

"Why did you wait so long to come and see us?" Nancy asked.

"It may be hard for you to understand why we waited about a year, but life was pretty good, and Missy never bugged me about it, did you, Missy? Also, I was able to get on social security disability, which paid actually more than my salary had been. So we were fine, and Missy was always around, and during the day, I listened to a lot of TV."

By now, the pupils had dilated, and Nancy could confirm that the patient had bilateral retinal detachments with multiple retinal holes.

A few minutes later, she came to get me to confirm her diagnosis, as she related the history to me. I then went on to explain what he had, in layman's terms.

"The retina is the inner lining in the back of the eye, like the inner tube of a bicycle. In your case, it developed some holes, so fluid, which fills up the eyeball, went through the holes and lifted up the retina, separating it from the next layer, the choroid, which is a vascular layer that supplies most of the oxygen and nutrients to the retina. The result is that the retina is no longer flat and is also not getting enough blood supply. Since the retina is the structure which does the seeing—that is, it is where the light coming into the eye through the pupil is focused—its lack of flatness prevents proper focusing, and its lack of nutrition makes it not work very well.

"Can this be fixed?" Missy asked.

"Yes, I think that we can reattach the retina surgically, but it is hard to guess how good your vision will be because you waited so long before coming to see us. Some of that retina has died by now, but you will, if we succeed, certainly see better than now. How much better, I just don't know, but the eye that went blind most recently has the best chance of some decent vision."

Joe spoke up, "Let's do it. The sooner the better."

"Are you sure, honey?" asked Missy.

"Yes, I'm sure. I shouldn't have waited this long."

"Okay. We'll schedule the first eye for next Tuesday. Nancy, why don't you get him ready for a scleral buckling procedure? Do a quick preop physical exam, a retinal drawing—you know the routine. And, Joe, I assume you have Medicaid?"

He nodded.

When Tuesday came, Joe was scheduled to be the second case. By 9:00 AM, he was ready to be wheeled into the OR. We transferred him from the stretcher to the operating table, but then he suddenly sat up with the announcement, "Sorry, Doc, but I can't go through with this. It's too scary."

"But yesterday, we got you all ready, and you signed the OR permit and seemed to be gung ho."

"Yeah, but last night, Missy talked me out of it. She's such a dear. She told me that it was no problem for her to take care of me. Now, I've got to get out of here. Let me get off this table."

"Are you absolutely sure?" the anesthetist asked.

"Yes, I've got to go. Please, please now!"

It seemed that Joe had made up his mind, and so we got him back on the stretcher and wheeled him out of the OR, transferred him to a wheelchair, and took him back to the waiting room, where we told Missy that the surgery was cancelled. She seemed relieved and smiled.

"I guess that he finally listened to me" was her comment.

I told her that I would call later because I needed to return to the OR, where I had three more cases to do. I looked at my watch. We had just wasted an hour.

During the next four weeks, I had several phone conversations with Missy and Joe and finally convinced them to go through with the surgery anyway.

"It's crazy to continue to be blind when there's a good chance that your vision will be improved. You still may not have great vision, but at least you'll be able to get around on your own."

A week later, we repeated the preop routine with the resident again doing an eye exam and a cursory physical exam to clear the patient for anesthesia. This time, we scheduled Joe as the last case of the day. My other cases went well, and by 3:00 PM, we were ready for Joe. We sent for the patient but were told that he and his wife were in the waiting room and wanted to talk to me. I found Missy and Joe sitting on a chair, with Joe still in his street clothes, obviously not ready for surgery.

"What is it this time, guys?" was my question.

Missy answered, "We just can't make up our minds. It's so hard, and we are not unhappy the way we are. And there is some risk, with the anesthesia and all."

Then Joe added, "I'm so sorry, but today is just not the day. I hope we didn't screw up your schedule too much."

"Well, I could have scheduled another case. So now the OR room is idle, and Anesthesia has nothing to do! All that costs money. The hospital doesn't like that. Why don't you just go home, think about it some more, and then call me? You have my number."

During the next few days, I discussed the situation with my office partner Dr. Raymond Stewart. He came up with a novel idea, agreeing with me that the patient definitely needed the operation, at least in one eye. He suggested that we ask the patient for money before his surgery. Then, if he changed his mind again, we would either keep the money or at least tell him that we would. However, if the patient went through with the surgery, we would give the money back and simply bill for the operation through Medicaid. I agreed to let Dr. Stewart call the patient to explain this scheme to him and also to convince Joe to go through with surgery after all. For Joe's sake, I surely hoped that Dr. Stewart would succeed where, apparently, I had failed. After several conversations, Joe and Missy seemed again convinced to try surgery and agreed to pay three hundred dollars up front.

For a third time, I put Joe on my schedule and asked the resident to confirm that the physical exam had not changed. This time, a senior medical student, rotating through Ophthalmology, was doing the physical exam to assure that the patient could be safely anesthetized. Being a medical student and learning about preop clearance, his exam was probably more thorough than was customary. He did the usual ENT check and listened to the heart and lungs to make certain that the patient had no upper respiratory infection and then palpated the abdomen, where he felt some resistance right under the breastbone. He pushed firmly to make sure that this was not just the liver, but this was different. This felt like a firm ball in an area that was normally soft and compressible. Not sure what to make of it, the student called me and asked if it was all right to get an internal medicine resident involved.

As it turned out, the student's exam was correct, and Joe was examined by several other physicians, who then ordered a series of blood tests as well as x-rays. It took ten days to come up with a diagnosis of probable pancreatic cancer, which had already spread to the liver and other abdominal organs. A fine-needle biopsy confirmed the diagnosis, and Joe was given the unhappy news that he might not survive for much more than a year. His condition was inoperable, and there was really no known treatment.

When I heard the news, I could hardly believe it. I had been so focused on his retinal detachments that the possibility of a second major medical disease in this relatively young person had not really occurred to me. It was certainly very unusual, but so was the whole situation. Never before had I had a patient refuse surgery for retinal detachment. Never before had I had a patient change his mind about surgery while he was already lying on the operating table. It was as if the patient somehow already knew that he did not need my surgical expertise.

During the next year, I stayed in touch with Joe, who started to become symptomatic from his metastatic disease. During his last few months, Missy took care of him with great apparent affection and without a single complaint.

Part V

ADJUSTMENTS

Chapter 1: Unrealized Potential 141
Chapter 2: Children 147
Chapter 3: Judgment 151
Chapter 4: Mamma Mia 159

Chapter 1

UNREALIZED POTENTIAL

Steve Fisher was a big man, more than six feet tall, weighing at least 250 pounds, and obviously very muscular. He was dressed in large baggy cargo pants, sneakers, and a T-shirt with the sleeves cut off, accentuating his biceps. But he looked pathetic, being led in by another man, shuffling his way along the hall into the exam room. The other man, who turned out to be his older brother, placed Steve's hands on the arms of the exam chair to help Steve sit down. It was obvious the patient could not see much.

The brother who was dressed in a shirt and tie gave most of the history. He himself had gone to college and become a librarian, but his younger brother had never wanted any education beyond high school. He had been fascinated early on by a summer job, during which he worked in construction and got to drive large machines, and so he became a bulldozer operator for a builder and specialized in digging house foundations and septic systems. But then he began having eye problems, episodes of painful red eyes and blurry vision accompanied by severe sensitivity to light. At first, he tried to hide his problem from his boss, wearing very dark sunglasses, which relieved his photophobia significantly and, at the same time, hid the redness of his eyes. But then, he backed his dozer into a dump truck, and at another time, he tipped over his own machine because he could not see well enough to judge the slope of the ground. The tip over almost killed him. He then had to take some time off but was back on the job two weeks later when his eye condition improved after taking some cortisone eye drops, which some pharmacist had given him.

During the next few months, he had several recurrences and was able to continue his job, but with several week-long interruptions. Each time that he went back to work, however, his vision was a little worse, and finally he was fired.

That was the moment when Jim, the brother, realized that he could play a role in Steve's life that he had never anticipated. Steve was not self-sufficient anymore, and Jim would become his caretaker. Their parents were old and sickly, living in a Medicaid nursing home and could not be helpful. Thus, the two brothers moved in together and were figuring out what the next steps should be just when Steve had another attack of painful redness and blurring. Jim, the academic, having faith in institutions of higher learning, decided to take Steve to the University, where he thought the likelihood of finding a treatment or cure was the greatest.

My examination was uncomfortable for Steve, because he really did not want to open his eyes, which seemed to hurt him a lot. The lights on the slit lamp and the ophthalmoscope were especially painful. Anesthetic drops did not help much, and so the exam went slowly. His vision was poor, although he could see light and motion, and the conjunctiva of both eyes was very inflamed. The corneal surface was normal, but behind it, in the anterior chamber of the eye, there was a lot of inflammatory debris, so I could barely see the blue color of his iris. The pupils, also hard to see, were constricted, thus not permitting me to see the lens or anything behind it. This was bilateral severe intraocular inflammation (anterior uveitis), but what was the cause? To relieve the spasm of the pupil, I instilled atropine eye drops, which, within a few minutes, relieved much of the pain. During these minutes, I could ask some more questions and also observe the entire patient a little more. I noticed that he had a habit of licking the inside of his lower lip, and so I asked him about that.

"Oh, I get these sores on my lips and in my mouth," he said as he everted his lip with his forefinger. "They come and go, usually stay about a week, and then they're gone. If it's on my lip, I use Blistex. If it's elsewhere in my mouth, I just use mouthwash. They come back every couple of months, but they don't bother me that much, although it sometimes hurts to eat when they are on my gums."

"Do these sores always happen at the same time that your eyes flare up?" "No, not always, but sometimes, like right now."

"Do you ever get these elsewhere?"

"What do you mean?" he asked nervously.

"Well, some people can get them on their penis or around their rear end."

He thought for a moment. "I may have had one on my foreskin some time ago. You know, I am not circumcised, but I never thought that it was the same kind of thing. Are you saying that this could be some venereal disease? That's impossible. I don't play around."

"No, I'm not suggesting that, not at all. But are there other infections you get, like on your skin or elsewhere?" That would help me figure out what you have."

He barely let me finish my sentence and pulled up one pants leg.

"I get these," and he rubbed his hand over his leg just below his knee. They looked like typical erythema nodosum lesions, one inch wide red (inflamed) bumps just below the kneecap.

"These really make my knees hurt."

This was my first time to see a patient with probable Behcet's disease. The classic triad was all there: bilateral uveitis, mucous membrane ulcers, and erythema nodosum in a young male. In a way, it was exciting to see an example of this disease, very rare in the United States but more common in Japan and Turkey. But at the same time, I felt sorry for Steve because there was really no known cure, and no one really knew much about Behcet or what caused it. I did tell him that specific attacks were often treatable with cortisone and assured him, pending a few blood tests, that I knew what he had and that we would be able to manage his problem.

He seemed relieved. During the next few days, I arranged for appointments with internal medicine and dermatology. Syphilis and sarcoidosis were ruled out, and the diagnosis was confirmed. Other than eye drops, steroid treatment was started, and a mild antimetabolite was added. The acute symptoms went away, leaving Steve with slightly diminished vision.

During the next few months, three things happened. First, there were two more recurrences, each time resulting in a further decrease in vision. The second was that Jim, the librarian brother, in his library research, learned that the National Eye Institute (NEI), part of the National Institutes of Health (NIH), was looking for patients with Behcet's disease for research purposes. The third was that Jim had finally convinced Steve to get more education and aim for a college degree. Jim told me that big boys don't need bulldozer toys anymore, and that it was time for Steve to grow up.

As a result, I called NEI saying that I had a Behcet patient. After hearing the details of Steve's case, they agreed. Jim drove Steve to Bethesda, Maryland, where he was admitted to the hospital for observation and testing. It was all free of charge and ended up lasting almost three months. Because Steve had so much free time while he was at the NEI and because he was not confined to a bed, he was able to spend many hours in the library. This had been suggested by Jim, who, through interlibrary loans, had created an entire curriculum for him to get him ready for college. A short phone call from me to the director of the NEI, who had been one of my mentors in medical school, resulted in making some magnifiers available to Steve so that his reading was facilitated.

When Steve came home to live with his brother again, his symptomatic episodes had decreased in frequency, and he was now on maintenance low-dose steroids and colchicine, a drug usually used to treat gout.

During the three months that Steve was away, Jim had been busy arranging for Steve's admission to the local community college. There was no question in his mind that this was the right thing to do, and so it happened.

Steve's college career went well, and he completed two years of work in sixteen months. Meanwhile, the occasional occurrence of his eye inflammation kept eroding his vision, and during the last two months, Jim had to help him daily with his studies. Steve could now barely see enough to walk in his own environment. To me, the reason for this visual decrease was not only the debris in the front of the eye but also because there was bleeding into the vitreous cavity of the eye, probably from the retina.

And so the studies were interrupted, and Steve, who had now been declared blind in the State of New York, was able to enroll in a free school for the blind, where he learned Braille, the tactile method of reading without using the eyes. He was a fast learner and could read fairly quickly just using his fingertips. Clearly Steve was a smart person and had become incredibly motivated to pursue book learning, with the enthusiastic support of his brother.

Special arrangements were now made at the college, which had never had a blind student before, but the administration saw it as a challenge. One and a half years later, Steve graduated with a major in business administration and a minor in education. He wanted to do something in the insurance business.

This timing coincided with the development of a new surgical technique, the vitrectomy, which was a way of removing tissue from the inside of the eye using a needle-like device that could be inserted through a small opening and could cut tissue, suck it out, and replace it with clear fluid. Steve seemed to be a good candidate for this procedure, since a major reason for his poor vision was debris and now blood inside the eyeball. I called around to several of my retina colleagues and also asked my Boston mentor for their opinions, but none had ever performed a vitrectomy on a Behcet patient.

The result of the operation in the first eye was amazingly good, and the bleeding vessels could be identified after the blood was removed. A subsequent laser treatment sealed the bleeders. Since the inflammatory episodes were now infrequent, there was no reason not to go ahead with a vitrectomy in the second eye. The result was similar, and the vision returned to 20/20. The elation of the two brothers was boundless. Naturally, I, too, was excited and relieved. It was like some sort of a miracle.

During the next two years, there were only three recurrences of the ocular inflammation, none of them with bleeding and all of them quickly contained with a temporary increase in medications. During that time, Steve travelled to NIH several times, resulting in a decrease in the medications needed. Still, however, the NEI did not know what exactly Behcet disease was, what caused it, why it occurred in some places in the world and not in others, and why there seemed to be no genetic pattern to it. It did run in families, however.

Then, during the next five years, when I continued to see Steve every few months, Steve's problem seemed to disappear, as so often happens in Behcet patients. When I last saw Steve, another ten years later, he was seeing well and had no more complaints. He was now the head of a small insurance agency in Upstate New York, had married, and had a small son. As a volunteer for the blind school, he taught Braille. He told me that anybody could only learn Braille well if they were really stone-blind.

Later, as I thought about Steve's story, I realized that his superhuman rapid mastery of Braille came at a time that he was highly motivated to get an education and that it was just one more hurdle to leap over. Nothing would have stopped him at that moment. All it took was motivation, a strong support system, and the promise of a better life to come. Anyone with those three elements in place, which doctors can often help provide, can probably achieve his or her potential, no matter how insurmountable the obstacles may seem.

Chapter 2

CHILDREN

Paulus Johannes Waardenburg, born in the Netherlands in 1886, studied science at the University of Utrecht some twenty years before my father studied medicine there and became immediately intrigued by genetics, long before much genetic information about human disease was known. Because Utrecht was, at that time, world famous in ophthalmology due largely to people like Donders and Snellen (the creator of the Snellen vision chart), it is understandable that Waardenburg's genetics interests focused on eye diseases and genetic blindness. There was plenty of material for him to study, as there seemed to be an unusually large number of visually impaired children in the country. Today, looking back, this may have been due to Holland's geography, which between 1860 and 1915, still consisted of many islands. Today it is connected by bridges but then only reachable by boat. It was a time of relative geographic isolation, which might have caused a certain amount of inbreeding, which, in turn, can lead to genetic combinations not often seen in less isolated areas.

Today, since the industrial revolution in the late 1800s and the electrification of Europe after 1900, this has all changed. Large dikes were constructed to connect islands, bridges were built elsewhere, water levels were controlled using new canals and sluices, and vast areas within dikes were pumped dry, often below sea level. Then a massive public transportation system, relying heavily on electric trains and trolleys, was created. All these modernizations changed Holland, made every corner of it easily accessible and eliminated the isolation problems.

In 1919, partly because of Waardenburg's interest in genetic blindness and his appointment as lecturer at the University at Utrecht, the Bartimeus School for blind children was started in a small town near the city. My father then became a regular consultant at that facility.

On some Saturdays, I, then about nine years old, would accompany him on his visits to the school that was housed in an old mansion and surrounded by several acres of well-manicured grounds, which consisted of several lawns, some large trees, and multiple white gravel paths which looped throughout the flat terrain. The perimeter was marked by a low fence with a metal bar on top, which was painted white in sharp contrast with the green surround.

While my father was inside the building talking to the administrator and one of the uniformed nurses who would take him to see one or more of the children, I was left outside in the park, where I could observe some of the children, who were running around and playing very similarly to the activity on any school playground. Had I not known better, I would never have suspected that these children were almost totally blind, even though some may have had light perception vision or even motion vision, so they may have been able to differentiate darkness from bright light, green grass from white paths, or gotten some sense of motion, if a large dark object moved in front of a bright background. I did know that, for children between six and fifteen, to be living or at least spending their days at the school, had to be virtually completely blind.

It was amazing to see the level of activity in the school park. Kids were running around playing tag while shouting at one another. Apparently, once you had been tagged, you had to shout out your name. There were also other sounds like the clapping of hands and the clicking noise of wooden castanets that some kids had in the palm of one hand. The speed of their running was astounding, considering the presence of some very large trees, which they were able to avoid. As they were running, shouting, clapping, and clicking, they frequently crossed one of the multiple graveled paths, which must have given them additional sensory input.

In one area, near the fence, some children swung on swings while others were paired up on several seesaws, and still others were climbing up a ladder to reach the top of a metal slide which ended up in a sand pit.

The most surprising performance I witnessed was the riding of bicycles on the gravelly paths. Clearly, they could hear the noise of their tires on the gravel and could also hear each other, but it seemed to me like a hazardous activity. It was little surprise when two children on bikes collided at the crossing of two paths. Obviously, the one child who was hit from the side was irritated and shouted at the other one as he was picking himself up from the ground, "Can't you watch where you're going?"

Neither child was hurt, and both got back on their bikes to continue their journeys.

As years went by and I myself entered ophthalmology, I was reminded many times of my Bartimeus experience. It became more and more clear that people with congenital blindness (blind from birth) need not be as devastated as one would think and can, with proper early intervention, schooling, and vocational training, lead happy and productive lives. I have had numerous blind patients—who came to me for eye infections, eyelid problems, or eye pain—who were successful and productive people, who were even married to fully sighted partners and had children. I have seen a blind insurance salesman, a blind psychologist, a blind president of a real estate company, and a blind woman, who was an international simultaneous translator and who was absolutely fluent in French, Italian, Spanish, and English.

In all these cases, it was early intervention by a Bartimeus-type institute that made the difference. I now often wonder what happened to the two boys who collided on their bikes. I am willing to wager that they are just fine.

Today, the Bartimeus Foundation is the largest organization providing services for the blind in the Netherlands, located at sixteen different locations throughout the country. It employs more than 2,000 and has almost 1,000 volunteers. They support 12,000 clients.

In the Western world, we are fortunate that many private and public organizations exist that have the same mission. In the United States, much like Bartimeus, private schools for the blind are scattered throughout the country. But in addition, every state has public programs for blind education. States know that if you give the blind educational opportunities, it ultimately saves money by keeping them off welfare. In addition, eye research, aimed at preventing blindness, is burgeoning, often supported by the National Eye Institute, part of the National Institutes of Health. It is hoped that those governmental agencies will continue to have the fiscal support from our political leaders. The private sector cannot do it alone.

Chapter 3

Judgment

Early in my academic career, as a junior faculty member in the late sixties, I had little to do with choosing which of the many applicants for our residency program we should interview. Our program was popular among East Coast graduates, and the more-than-two-hundred applications for four positions gave us some assurance that whomever we picked would be well qualified. The chairman usually made a list of about forty of the best applicants for personal interviews, which were scheduled in the fall of each year, ten interviews a day every Friday for about a month. That's where I got involved, as did the rest of the faculty. Each of us ranked the applicants according to their credentials and personality, and then, during a faculty meeting, often lasting more than three hours, a master list would be agreed upon. The applicants also made their own list of programs where they had been granted interviews, and the "match" occurred late in the fall. Years later, this match, originally done manually, was computerized, minimizing the chance of error.

One of our residents, who had survived this vetting process because of the stellar recommendations from his medical school mentors, was a delightful young man named Steve, with reddish hair and freckles, good-looking, tall, and with a disarming personality. It was very easy to like him instantly, which translated into a good bedside manner. One middle-aged patient, a beautiful and energetic woman, once told me, after meeting Steve, that she wanted to put him in her pocket and take him home.

Toward the end of Steve's first of his three years of residency, I began to notice that he occasionally looked walleyed, not with his eyes crossed inwardly but with one eye drifting outward. It was most noticeable at the end of a day, presumably because he was tired. I mentioned it to our chairman, a pediatric ophthalmologist, who was going to look into it. This was the first time we heard Steve's eye history, how he was cross-eyed as a small child, had been treated with glasses since kindergarten, and then was finally operated at age seven to improve his appearance, since other children in school were ridiculing him. It was not an uncommon story for congenital strabismus (crossed eyes), and the surgery made him look normal, although he never developed good vision in one eye. Therefore, he never had good stereoscopic vision but managed just fine in ordinary life, since he did not know what he was missing. He was simply one of the 10 percent of Americans with good vision in one eye only. He mentioned that his eye problem had given him a special interest in ophthalmology and was probably the reason why he chose it.

During the next six months, his exotropia (outward eye deviation) became more obvious, and Steve wondered whether more could be done for cosmetic reasons. He didn't think that an eye doctor should have an obvious eye problem that patients could see. The chairman agreed and, under local anesthesia, in the operating room, performed a surgical adjustment of his eye muscles, with a wonderful cosmetic result. The eyes were now again well aligned, although the vision in one eye was still poor and was expected to remain so for life.

At one of the faculty meetings, we discussed Steve's situation and questioned how his monocular (one-eyed) vision would impact his training, particularly now that he was starting to learn eye surgery. Without true depth perception, would he really be able to judge very small distances within the eye and know how close the instrument tips were to vital structures, such as the lens or the retina? Was it possible for someone who had never had 3D vision to have developed

THE EYE: WINDOW TO BODY AND SOUL

enough visual experience to make these judgments based on size of object, movement, or some other learned visual experience? Then there was the fact that most eye exam tools were now binocular, such as the slit lamp, ophthalmoscope, and operating microscope. Every time that one of these had gone from being monocular to binocular, it had been a breakthrough for the ophthalmic practice, facilitating more precise diagnoses and surgery. We decided that we would watch Steve very closely as he learned our profession.

To our surprise, he did not seem to be hampered by his handicap, especially during surgery. In fact, he learned cataract surgery easily and even excelled in it. We were all relieved and stopped worrying about the possibility that we would graduate an ophthalmic surgeon who was visually impaired. There was, however, one concern that arose only a few times, when, on his senior rotation on the retina service, he was asked to draw the retina of patients in preparation for retinal surgery, usually the repair of retinal holes, tears, or retinal detachments. He was simply not as good as most residents at identifying the pathology. This didn't worry us much, since he planned to be a general ophthalmologist, and they did not perform retina surgery. The student would have to take an additional one or two years of a retinal fellowship to do that, and Steve had no such plans.

After Steve graduated, he returned to his hometown, some thirty miles away, to start a solo practice, which blossomed quickly, since he was the only ophthalmologist in that community and was also a native son. People in town were very pleased that he had returned home. We also were happy that he remained in the area so that we could continue to stay in touch. We saw him regularly at some of our grand rounds or whenever we had a visiting lecturer. He also periodically referred patients for subspecialty care, such as complex glaucoma or retina surgery.

On two occasions, within one month, we saw two of his patients, both in their midforties, because they had each developed retinal tears (holes) at an unusually early age. The first of these, a fair-haired, pale-skinned yoga teacher apparently had four or five horseshoe-shaped tears in each eye, which he had treated with laser. The second was another blue-eyed blonde with similar findings. He had not treated her pending our opinion whether or not she should be treated. Horseshoe tears were precursors to retinal detachment, and he had been taught by us to treat them, even if they were not accompanied by the usual symptoms of flashes or floaters. When I saw the first patient and examined the retina, the laser scars were obvious in the midperiphery of the retina in both eyes. However, I could not see any evidence of retinal holes in the center of the laser scars. Instead, the treatment seemed to have been in the area of the vortex veins, the large collecting veins draining the circulation underneath the retina, which were very visible in this light-skinned patient. In a darker-skinned patient, the pigment layer between the mostly transparent retina and the vascular layer (choroid) would have been more developed and hidden the vessels from view. Could it have been that Steve misinterpreted the shape of these bright-red sharply delineated veins for retinal tears?

I called him to say that I saw no other retinal pathology and that further treatment was not needed. I also assured him that his light laser treatment would not have done any damage to the venous circulation.

When the second patient came, I was prepared. She brought with her a retinal drawing which Steve had given her. He obviously wanted to show off that he had not forgotten his training on the retinal service. The drawing showed multiple tears in the midperipheral retina of both eyes in the exact location of the vortex veins. Clearly the edge of each vein was indeed shaped like the typical horseshoe tear and was even the approximate size of such a typical tear. I again called Steve and thanked him for the referral. I told him about my findings and mentioned that his drawing was appreciated and gave me the opportunity to look very carefully at his areas of concern.

"I am absolutely sure that there are no holes or tears in the retina, and what you have drawn are the vortex veins. I must admit that they are horseshoe-shaped and also the right size to make one think they may be retinal pathology, but in this case, the retinas are okay.

Thanks for the referral. Keep them coming!" I laughed and switched the conversation to other subjects. I told him the department was doing well and that our newly selected residents were from all over the country, including California, Utah, and Michigan. That was certainly different than in the old days, when most applicants were from New York City or at least from New York State. He told me that his practice was busy and varied, with more ophthalmic plastic surgery than he had anticipated. In the previous year, he had taken a special course at the American Academy just to brush up on how to deal with all those droopy eyelids. It was a very pleasant and friendly discussion, which gave me the chance to ask a special question.

"By the way, Steve, you just made me think of something. Do you think that your having only one good eye made it more difficult to judge whether it was a vortex vein or a tear that you were looking at?"

"I dunno" was his quick reply. We ended the conversation with a few more pleasantries and my final comment: "Stay in touch!"

During the following months, the number of retinal referrals seemed to increase, and each time the patient brought a retinal drawing along.

Then, during one of our faculty meetings, my story about Steve was discussed, and a decision was made to request that each resident applicant submit an ophthalmologist-signed eye exam document, indicating best-corrected visual acuity and proof of stereoscope vision.

Many years later, when I became chairman of another department, this subject arose again. I had frankly forgotten about Steve's story. One year, as I was sorting through the many applications to determine which candidates should be interviewed, there was one applicant photo unlike any other. It was a profile photo rather than the usual full-face image. Other than noticing this fact, I thought nothing further of it. The candidate was from Pittsburgh, where his father was an ophthalmologist, and had excellent credentials and recommendations. I picked him to be interviewed.

On the Friday that he came, he was one of twelve. It was going to be a busy day, with each student being interviewed by six faculty members. I was the second person to meet with him and immediately noticed, as he sat across the desk from me, that his eyes were not aligned. My first question therefore was about his vision.

"How good is your vision?"

"Excellent, 20/20 with my glasses."

"No, I mean your vision in each eye. I want to know what you can see out of your left eye, which is not looking straight at me."

"It's not as good as the right, but . . . pretty good."

"Well, what is it? Do you know, or do we have to test it?"

"I think it's about 20/200."

"How long have you had one bad eye?"

"Since I was a kid. I was cross-eyed, and my father operated on me and straightened it out."

"How old were you then?"

"I think about four. I don't really remember."

"I just want you to know that I am not going to continue to interview you. No one else will be meeting with you either. My suggestion is that you pack up your stuff, go to the airport, and go home. We will not be ranking you because the department does not train residents unless they have good vision in each eye and good stereo vision."

"But it doesn't say that, or anything about that, in your brochure."

"I am sorry, but that's the way it is."

He left angrily, murmuring some expletive under his breath.

A few hours later, I got an angry phone call from his father. How could I treat his son so badly? He was going to make sure that no one from Pittsburgh would ever apply to our program again. He was going to sue us. After his tirade, I told him about Steve and that it should be obvious to any ophthalmologist that practicing without good vision in both eyes could be dangerous for patients. I did admit that it was an oversight on my part not to have mentioned binocularity as a prerequisite for incoming residents. My apology calmed him down somewhat, and we agreed that I would reimburse his son for his airline expenses. I did point out, however, that his son had clearly tried to hide his visual handicap by submitting a photo taken from the side.

I also added, "Sir, do you really think that it is fair to push your son towards ophthalmology? I also am the son of an ophthalmologist, so I understand how much pressure, even unknowingly, a father can exert on the career choice of a son. But does it have to be a surgical subspecialty? How about some branch of medicine that does not require stereo vision?"

At the next faculty meeting, when we discussed the interviewees, we had a lively discussion formalizing a list of requirements for potential residents. One faculty member told the story of a navy heart surgeon, with poor vision in at least one eye, who was convicted of involuntary manslaughter and negligent homicide due to technical incompetence, because of his vision problem, which he had hidden. He was jailed but later released from prison because the evidence seemed insufficient. We all agreed that we would not want that to happen to any of our graduates. Another faculty member suggested that we demand a complete exam, maybe even a complete physical exam and medical history, signed by an MD. At the end of the meeting, I promised to get advice from some national leaders in ophthalmology.

At first, I spoke to the president of the AUPO, the Association of University Professors in Ophthalmology, an organization whose members were all the chairpersons of ophthalmology departments across the country. He informed me that there was no national policy and that most departments had never had to deal with this issue.

"Don't you think there should be a policy?

His answer was humorous.

"Right now, I can think of at least three chairmen who are monocular. There may be more. In each of these cases, they had good binocular vision earlier in their careers, and now none of them operates any more. But still, I think the suggestion of creating a policy wouldn't go very far with them."

Then, I called the president of the AAO, the American Academy of Ophthalmology. He had actually heard about other instances where binocularity had been questionable in some resident candidates. He felt that each program could set its own standards and make that known to applicants as they were deciding where to apply. That would certainly avoid any lawsuits, as long as the requirements were not too overreaching or unreasonable. He agreed with me that good vision, with or without glasses; stereo vision; and normal color vision were reasonable requirements. Then he warned me not to perform those tests ourselves but to let each candidate, with their application, submit the results of these tests, signed by an ophthalmologist.

When I took these recommendations to our faculty, we all agreed that we would follow that advice. Since then, the issue has not arisen in the department, but we are all watchful for signs of poor clinical judgment and hope that it will never be due to something like uncorrectable poor vision.

Chapter 4

Mamma Mia

She was a woman of great conviction, whom I knew well. The only daughter of a tall, strong, silent, and proud father of Nordic birth, who had left the family farm to become a dentist in the city, she was brought up in her daddy's image to be self-reliant, confident, and educated. A leader among her classmates at Utrecht University in Holland, she studied law and became a judge. She then married a physician and produced two sons, who benefitted from her strength, especially during the war years in the forties.

When the family moved to the United States after the war, tired of turmoil and hoping to find a better and more stable future for the boys, her strength helped find direction and stability in this new land.

In the sixties, her husband died, and she moved to an apartment overlooking the ocean across which she had come. She had never really become an American, although she did have her US citizenship, and had retained strong opinions, feelings, and habits from her youth. God forbid she should miss her afternoon tea with cookies!

In the eighties, her arthritis got the best of her. She had always been tall and heavy, weighing 180 pounds—big boned, she called it—which finally took its toll on her knees and hips. Walking became difficult, and nursing help became necessary. She was moved to a nearby nursing home, which she seemed to enjoy at first, because she was mentally alert, pleased with her tea in the afternoon, able to reread all her books she had kept from her younger years, and willing to expound to the staff and other patients about Europe, the war, moving to America, and about her sons.

She was eighty-one when her glasses were lost. At first, she complained bitterly while the staff looked in vain through her room and laundry to find them. After two weeks, however, she seemed not to care whether she had them or not and also appeared to lose some interest in her environment, an understandable phenomenon in any uncorrected myope, who cannot see at distance. Of course, she could not see herself in the mirror either. Thus stopped the eighty-year-old ritual of combing the hair before breakfast. On some days, she even neglected to put in her dentures, which suddenly made her face look sunken and ancient—again, not seen by her. She also stopped reading, an activity so dear to her, for which she needed glasses. Food also became uninteresting, and she essentially stopped feeding herself. The nursing staff would try to feed her, often with great difficulty, as she clenched her mouth tightly shut. She lost seventy pounds.

An effort was made to get her refracted. Machine-hoisted out of bed on a sling, placed on her wheelchair, then put in the van to the ophthalmologist's office, she refused to cooperate, did not wish to look through the phoropter, and shook her head to get rid of the trial frame. A pair of glasses was prescribed, which, by estimate, gave her 20/30 vision. She never used them.

I started to wonder. Had the loss of her glasses suddenly so isolated her from her environment that all the stimuli, cues, and distractions that keep us going were gone? The timing was certainly right! Her downhill course had started immediately following the loss of glasses. Or was it simply time to quit? Being a person whose destiny was always in her own hands, she had once made the remark that she only wanted to live until eighty-two, the age at which her father had died. Eighty-two was now!

She died a few weeks later. Her pulse had been slow and strong up to the very end. Her death certificate stated cardiopulmonary arrest (no disease) as the cause. It might have stated "loss of glasses."

Part VI

ARE THEY CRAZY?

Chapter 1: Afraid 163
Chapter 2: Give Me a Break 170

Chapter 1

AFRAID

Florence Fitzgerald had always been involved with schools, first as a teacher in fifth and sixth grade and later as principal of an elementary school and, subsequently, a high school. She was married briefly, had two children, and got divorced, impatient with the arrogant ineptitude of men, as she put it. On the side, she earned enough money to live in one of the best neighborhoods in town, where the public school system was excellent. She was a no-nonsense person, strict with her children but provided a nurturing environment for them, which emphasized education. She always read to them when they were young and always found games for them to play, which required some use of mathematics. Crossword puzzles were a weekly routine. So was church. Never would the three of them miss Sunday Mass, and both children sang in the choir. It was little surprise that both ended up going to the University of Texas School of Law in Austin, ranked as one of the best in the country, and both became judges.

As Florence approached seventy, she came to my office, referred by another ophthalmologist because of macular degeneration. She was now no longer a school principal but had expanded her tax work and was the CEO of a tax accounting firm. She had driven herself because her vision, at least in one eye, was still good. In the waiting room, she was the best-dressed person—her slightly graying russet hair clipped close to her head with a boyish part on one side, and she wore a dark-blue business suit, a beautiful color combination. Her pocketbook was a briefcase.

"I'm here because of macular degeneration," she said. "Several of my friends from Alamo Heights go to you as well for the same reason, so I want to know if I have it or not. You apparently know something about it."

"A little. Why don't I take a look?"

She proceeded to give me her medical history. There was little to tell except for a quick scare years before with a lump in her breast, which was removed and proved to be a stage I cancer. She was fine ever since. That was twenty years ago. Right now, she was healthy and only took an occasional Colace for constipation and a nasal spray during the allergy season in the spring.

"I'm as young and energetic as my kids," she said.

The examination was quick, only interrupted by a ten-minute wait while her pupils dilated, which always happens more quickly in blue-eyed persons. Everything looked normal except for the earliest signs of cataract in both eyes and some pigment mottling in the center of each retina, the macula. The latter could explain why her vision was 20/70 in the right eye and 20/30 in the left. She was unable to see the 20/20 line with either eye but would still be able to drive legally, since worse than 20/40 with both eyes open was the legal cutoff in Texas.

"You do have some very early cataract opacities in both your lenses, but that is not affecting your vision right now. In fact, if you ever in your lifetime develop significant lens problems, it will be many years from now, and at that time, cataract surgery can always be done. What is significant now is an area in the center of both retinas, in the macular area, that has some pigment shifting going on. The pigment, in a very important layer under the retina, is moving around, clumping together in certain areas, and has caused some depigmented areas adjacent to the clumps. The question now is whether this is just an aging change or the beginning of a degenerative change that will affect your vision. First, let's see if we can improve your vision with a prescription change in your glasses. Then, we will take some pictures of the retina for future reference so I can see during the next few months if things are changing. Then, let's do some fluorescein angiography, where we inject some fluorescein dye into an arm vein and see if the dye leaks out in the macular area, which we can photograph. That would help me differentiate so-called wet, with a leak, from dry macular degeneration, where there is no leak. We can do all this right now, and then we'll talk."

I called for the technician to pick her up.

"See you in about forty minutes."

She stood up briskly and followed the tech out the door. About an hour later, I had my answers. Her vision could be improved to 20/20 in the left eye but could not be improved in the right with any different prescription. The photographs demonstrated that the depigmentation of the right was precisely central, while similar depigmentation in the left was off-center with the very center being spared. The angiography showed no leakage, so this was not wet degeneration, which might be treatable with a laser burn.

I explained the situation to her and recommended that she take a special multivitamin with zinc, which some studies had shown to slow down further degeneration.

"I'm sorry that, at this time, there is no definitive treatment for what you have, but the vitamins should help, and let's pray for some luck."

"Yes, let's do that, but I'm doing just fine right now. I'll also keep my fingers crossed."

During the next six months, I saw her twice, just for reassurance. At the second visit, she was half an hour late for her appointment, because, she laughed, she had driven to the grocery store by mistake instead of to my office.

"Sometimes, I'm just a little forgetful," she said.

"Last week, I got into my car to go somewhere, but by the time I got to my car, I couldn't remember where I was going. That was actually the second time that happened."

"Do you forget other things, like names of people or places?"

"No, not usually."

"How about what day or month it is?"

"Sometimes."

"Do you pay your own bills and keep track of your own business accounts?"

"Oh, yes. I'm right on top of that. I'm very good with numbers."

During the next two years, Florence experienced a slight noncorrectable decrease in vision in both her eyes. It was very gradual, so that she either did not or pretended not to notice. She kept driving, and her business was doing well. She came to our office twice a year. Then, during the next five years, her vision decreased significantly. She was no longer driving and instead was dropped off at her office every day by her daughter. She still ran her business but had several assistants for the detailed paperwork. She carried a pocket magnifying glass and had a large desktop magnifier for documents. A lot of her time was spent interviewing clients. Few people recognized her handicap, although some of her closer friends did notice her sporadic forgetfulness and the occasional conversation she would start and then was unable to complete. She had also begun to talk about her dreams, which frequently centered around people whom she really could not remember ever meeting, but they were very nice and she would ski or sail with them or else take walks in the Swiss mountains.

At this visit, I told Florence that I was glad she was not driving anymore, because I was really obliged to let the motor vehicle department know about her legal blindness. I also repeated, as usual, the eye exam and the angiogram, the latter to confirm that her degeneration had not become wet.

As she was having this test performed by a technician, I had a chance to speak with the daughter.

"My brother and I are really quite worried about Mom," she told me. "She puts up quite a front, but we know that she's having real problems. She even got lost the other day in our own neighborhood. One of her friends saw her wandering around and took her home, but she couldn't tell me who that friend was—only that it was a man whom she knew quite well—she just couldn't think of his name, and she wasn't lost. She was following a bunch of very nice people who seemed to be going to a party. Both my brother and I think that she is losing it and should probably be moved to an elderly care facility. She just refuses and keeps insisting that she is fine. And then there are these dreams. She had never ever mentioned dreams before. Sometimes I think that they are not really dreams, but she really believes these things are happening. Is she going crazy?"

When Florence came back from her tests and I saw the results, I could assure both of them that the macular degeneration had not become wet and that we would simply continue with the vitamins, but then I lied to the daughter, saying, "Why don't we do a couple of more tests so I can be doubly sure of what I am saying? It may take another hour or so. Don't you have something else to do in the meantime?"

"Yes, I could go for a quick shop."

"Why don't you do that? We'll be here when you get back."

The daughter left, giving me a chance to ask Florence a few more questions. There were really no other tests I wanted to do. I just needed to explore an idea that had occurred to me.

"Tell me more about your dreams. Are they really dreams at night, or do they happen during the day as well?"

"Yes, they can occur during the day sometimes."

"Even when you are not taking a nap?"

"Yes, they can happen any time. They come on quite suddenly, and they go away suddenly too."

"Are they really dreams, or are they really . . . hallucinations? Are you seeing things? Are these things you have experienced before?"

She hesitated.

"I guess you could call them hallucinations," she said, and then quickly she added, "But don't tell my daughter because she'll really think I am nuts, and she will want to lock me up in a nursing home. That scares me. The hallucinations, the things I see, do not scare me at all. In fact, during these episodes, I really feel quite calm. What I see are faces, a group of people's faces who are very pleasant, very nice, with whom I'd like to be friends. And then they disappear. Sometimes, I even look forward to seeing them again."

"You know, Florence," I said, holding her hand, "you have just described something that is quite common in people who have lost a lot of vision. It is called Charles Bonnet syndrome and was first described more than one hundred years ago by a French ophthalmologist, whose grandfather had this condition. It has nothing to do with your mind, nothing to do with any medical illness, nothing to do with your mental capacity. You are not going crazy. You are not psychologically losing it. It only has to do with poor vision due to an eye condition. Your brain is simply trying to put some images together to make up for having lost visual stimulation from your eyes. You have nothing to worry about. You just need to know that you have Charles Bonnet syndrome, and you should tell people that."

I waited a few moments to let all this sink in.

"In fact, let me tell your daughter, and also your son, what is going on. Once they understand that this happens all the time in people with poor vision, they'll realize that you are not losing it, not going crazy. They'll stop threatening you with the nursing home. Do you have any friends with macular degeneration?"

"Yes, I have two good friends who see as poorly as I do, even worse."

"Well, talk to them and see if they have experienced the same thing. You may be surprised. Most people don't like to talk about it, because they are afraid, just like you, that people will think they are demented or crazy."

I laughed. "They don't want to be locked up either."

When Florence's daughter returned, I told her that we had not really done any more tests but that her mother had a classic case of Charles Bonnet syndrome. I gave her a brief summary of the condition, which our secretary had pulled off the computer and suggested she share that with her brother. I also gave her a website address where she could find out more.

Following that encounter, there seemed to be a new understanding between Florence and her children. They stopped threatening her with a nursing home and instead found her a retired schoolteacher, who was happy with room and board and a small weekly stipend. Florence also stopped talking about her dreams. Instead, whenever the subject arose, she would proudly and without fear announce to her friends, family, doctors, and anyone else who would listen, "I'm doing just fine. I do have some problems with my vision, and I have Charles Bonnet syndrome."

Chapter 2

GIVE ME A BREAK

The father of one of my close friends was always complaining about his vision and not knowing which of his many glasses to wear for what he was doing. His family had stopped driving with him because of his upsetting behavior with comments like, "I can't see a goddamn thing. I can't read those signs, can you?" "Are you sure we are on route 108? I never saw the sign." "Do you have any idea what the speed limit is?" "Help me put some gas in this car. I can't read what the pump is asking me to do." "Do they want the zip code now?" His wife had noticed that, while driving, he frequently wore different glasses on different days. Then, at home, he had glasses everywhere, some seeming to work better than others for whatever activity he was doing at the time. Some were glasses from before his first cataract operation, others for the time between cataract operations, and then he had several pairs given to him by a Costco optometrist in their vision center after both cataracts had been done. Being impatient and not thinking much of optometrists anyway, he had also bought some reading glasses of various strengths at the drugstore, whenever he saw a nice-looking frame.

Mr. Samuels had finally been convinced by his son to see me to explain about different glasses. He hadn't seen me since his son and I were high school classmates, so it was hard for him to believe that I had actually learned something since then. It was now almost twenty years later. To convince him, his son had mentioned that I was now an associate professor at the medical school, so I must know something.

Mr. Samuels was accompanied by his wife, a soft-spoken small woman with an empathetic demeanor, someone resilient enough to neutralize her husband's brusque personality. He preceded her into the exam room and sat down.

"Nice to see you again, Wick. I guess it's been awhile. I can't believe that you've actually grown up."

He smiled, finding himself amusing. Then, turning to his wife, he said, "Isn't it amazing, hon? He's a real doctor." With that comment, he reached into his pocket and pulled out a handful of spectacles, nine in all, and placed them on the table. "Here, Doc, you figure it out. Tell me which ones I should wear."

"Let me get some help with this. First, I want you to see our optometrist, just down the hall, to check on what distance prescription you really need, if any. While you do that, let me get your eye history from your wife, and we'll go from there."

After he left, I heard the whole story. Several years before, he had started to complain of glare. At night, he had trouble driving because the oncoming headlights blinded him. During the day, he could see well, 20/20 according to his eye doctor, but he started to wear sunglasses more often on bright days, especially in winter after a snowfall. He had been told that he had early cataracts but that it was too soon to operate. Unless the opacities in his lenses became intolerable, cataract surgery was not indicated yet. That then happened during the next two years. He complained more and more bitterly, unwilling to admit that a healthy guy like him had anything wrong. He had already been through the whole mess of needing increasingly strong reading glasses during his forties, as the elasticity of his lenses diminished and near focusing became more difficult. That in itself was an unwelcome reminder of the aging process. And now this! It made him very frustrated, she said.

When Mr. Samuels returned to the exam room, he finished telling the rest of his history. A year ago, after increasing complaints, he convinced his ophthalmologist to do one cataract operation in his worst eye, even though the vision was barely decreased (20/30), but his light sensitivity was almost constant, like having a dirty windshield in your car, which you only notice on a bright day or with oncoming headlights at night. He now wore polarized sunglasses even inside the house. And so one cataract operation was done. The lens in the eye was replaced by a plastic lens, which was intended to give him close to excellent vision at distance, with the understanding that, for any near task, he would need some glasses correction. The optical power of that correction would be different depending on how close things were that he wanted to see. There had been a long discussion about the different near tasks he usually performed. For reading at approximately one-third of a meter, the customary reading distance, he would need a three-diopter reading glass. If his computer screen was farther away at about half a meter, he would require a less powerful lens of two diopters. If the distance between his eye and his dashboard fuel gauge or speedometer was even greater than that, an even weaker lens would be needed. He was warned that he might, therefore, need several different pairs of glasses, one of which would always be in his car, one next to his computer, and still another for golf. And if his distance vision wasn't perfect without a prescription, these glasses might all be bifocals. He said the discussion almost drove him crazy. After the operation, his vision was decidedly better, as was his light sensitivity, but he was not happy with the temporary new glasses he got while waiting for the second eye to be operated. He was now wearing three different bifocals, but he felt dizzy at times and even saw double once in a while, which was particularly bothersome looking at the yellow line separating lanes of traffic. And so a few months later, partly because of his poor adjustment to his new glasses, he had the second cataract operation. Again, his vision improved slightly, but now his glare was completely gone. A few weeks later, when his vision had stabilized and he was no longer taking his postoperative eye drops, he revisited the optician with great hopes for ocular comfort. He said that he was in a great mood and got new eyeglass frames, which made him look younger.

Unfortunately, the optician talked him into progressive lenses, which were "the latest" and "the way to go." It was explained that these lenses were ground in such a way that the top of each lens would have the small distance prescription and that the bottom would be for reading.

From top to bottom, there would be a gradual increase in optical power so that he could always focus on anything at any distance, depending on what part of the lens he looked through.

"It was a disaster," Mr. Samuels said. "Here I spend three hundred dollars for a new frame, then another hundred or more for progressive lenses, and everything I looked at was crooked. It was all distorted! I didn't know what part of the lens to look through! I think the guy just wanted to make more money instead of giving me regular bifocals with a line between the top and the bottom of the glass. Everybody knows I am over forty, so I don't care if people see that line in my glasses."

When he had finished talking, he reached into his coat pocket and gave me the glasses again. This time each pair was in a little plastic baggie with a small yellow Post-it note attached, on which the optometrist had written the prescription. In addition, there was a note from the optometrist indicating that for distance, the patient only needed a very weak prescription in each eye, meaning that Mr. Samuels could probably see quite well without any distance prescription at all.

"Well, it looks like your cataract surgeon did a great job, just what you asked for. He hit the numbers just right. Your distance prescription is almost zero. You should be able to see pretty well without any glasses. Isn't that true?"

"Yes, but not if I want to read."

"Sure, but we'll talk about that later. First though, let me do a quick eye exam to make sure everything else is all right."

"Do I really need that? I just want you to sort out my glasses, that's all." "I would be remiss if I didn't do the whole exam."

"Let him do his thing," his wife suggested. "Okay, I guess."

The exam was quick. His pupils, less reactive following the cataract surgery, did not have to be dilated to give me a good intraocular view. The only abnormal finding was nicking of the retinal blood vessels, a narrowing of the veins where the small arteries crossed, indicating arteriosclerosis.

"Mr. Samuels, do you have high blood pressure?" "I was told that."

"Do you take anything for that?"

"I'm supposed to, but it doesn't seem to do anything. It doesn't make me feel any better."

"Let me first take your blood pressure, if you don't mind. It'll just take a minute." He stuck out his arm as I put the cuff around it. The pressure was 164/110.

"Your pressure is quite high, and it's probably been that way for quite a while. I can see it in your retina. Did you take your pressure pill today?"

"No, I haven't taken it for months. Maybe I don't need it. You're just making me nervous, that's why my pressure is high right now."

"I don't think so. This has been going on for maybe years. Otherwise I wouldn't see it in your retina. Do you mind if I call your general doctor about it so he can see you fairly soon?"

Then, turning to his wife, I asked her, "Could you make sure he gets an appointment? Uncontrolled high blood pressure can really do some damage, like a heart attack or a stroke."

"I'll take care of it," she stated firmly.

"Everything else looks all right, though. So now, let's talk about your glasses. These three here are no good anymore. They must've been from before your cataract surgery. The frames are also old and bent. Just put them aside. Then there are these two, which were possibly the ones you got between your first cataract operation and the second one. They are both bifocals, as you can see, and the bottom section is for reading at a +3.00 in one and a +2.50 in the other. This second one is more for the computer. But the top prescription is only good for the right eye, not for the left. Did you have your right eye done first?"

"Yes, that's right."

"Let me give these to your wife. The frames look new and are in pretty good shape. If you ever want to use these, you could always get the second lens replaced. That would be cheap. Then there are two more here. These are progressive lenses. They don't look like bifocals, they have no line, but if you hold them up to the light and look through them, you can see that the bottom of each lens is stronger than the top. You don't need these. You didn't like progressives. Why do you have two pairs?"

"The second one was half price."

"Well, one of these frames was the one you really liked and cost you so much. Why not keep that frame and then have your regular bifocal prescription put into it? Why don't we mark the Post-it note suggesting that you can do this later? Then there are two more pairs of glasses here. Both of them are fine for now. Both are bifocals, both for perfect distance vision, this one for reading, and this other one for the computer or the car. I suggest you mark them with colored nail polish at the end of one arm of the frame. Mark the reading one, which starts with an *R*, with red nail polish. If your computer is silver colored, mark this other one with silver nail polish. In fact, I would do this with all your glasses. What color is your car?"

"Sort of blue."

"Then mark your car glasses with blue polish. I know this works really well. My wife does this."

His wife spoke up. "I can do that!"

"Are we finished with this?" I asked.

"Almost." He reached into his other pocket and, to my amazement, pulled out four more pairs of glasses and plopped them on the table.

"What about these?"

I hesitated briefly. I wasn't sure whether I wanted to continue playing this game. Should I send him back to the optometrist to check on the power of the lenses? As I looked at the glasses, it quickly became apparent that these were all drugstore glasses of various powers, with the strength of the glasses printed on the inside of one arm.

"These are readers of various strengths. Remember +3.00 or +2.50 is for reading. The strength +2.00 is for the computer. The strength +1.00 is for golf. Just have your wife mark them with nail polish. My wife's golf glasses are painted white, like a golf ball."

"I think that does it," I said, relieved. "Just make sure that you make an appointment with your doctor. Don't forget! I'll also call him. It's Jason Carter, isn't it?"

He nodded.

"Well, Mr. and Mrs. Samuels, it's been a pleasure to see both of you. Please give my best to your son. I hope that you got your glasses sorted out."

As I was finishing my sentence, Mrs. Samuels was rummaging through her oversized bag. She looked up at me, seemingly having found what she was looking for.

"Dr. van Heuven, I almost forgot. What about these?" she asked, and she carefully placed four more pairs of glasses on my table.

Part VII

THE DOCTOR PERSEVERES

Chapter 1: The Graduate 179
Chapter 2: Iron Lady 186
Chapter 3: Elite 193

Chapter 1

THE GRADUATE

Sally McDonald first came to our office when she was in her late sixties, having heard that our Department of Ophthalmology was involved with eye research. Many years earlier, she had been told that she had drusen of the macula, small deposits under the central retina which could lead to macular degeneration. She remembered how her own father, a Baptist minister in a small town in the Texas Hill Country just north of Austin, had struggled with poor vision late in his life. It made preparing his sermons difficult, and many times, Sally would help him read and then write out the outline of the Sunday message in large letters. It had always amazed her how he had been able, from just those few large words on a page, to deliver a beautiful, unfaltering speech, quoting the Bible from memory, not letting his congregation even suspect his reading disability.

Sally had been referred by a classmate of her daughter's husband, a young urologist who had been trained at our University of Texas medical school in San Antonio. He had heard about our research and knew about Sally's intellectual curiosity.

When she arrived at the office, she had immediately asked for my educational credentials. When she heard the names of the Ivy League schools I had attended, she told the receptionist, "Well, that's good. I, too, went East for my education."

She had driven the eighty miles to San Antonio herself, using a GPS system that was brand-new at the time. She loved the latest technology. She was always fascinated by new discoveries, unlike many of her friends who wanted nothing to do with modern gadgets. They didn't even own computers. She told me why she came to see us, even though she really had no special vision problems at the moment.

"I was told years ago, when I started needing reading glasses, that I had drusen. I did some computer research and found out that some types of drusen can lead to macular degeneration. I certainly don't ever want that. I think my father had that." She then proceeded to tell me how she helped him with his sermons.

"I still have things to do. You know, I never got my college degree. Daddy sent me to a great school in the East, Bryn Mawr, but it was only a two-year college. Then I came home, got married to Seth McDonald of the McDonald ranch not far from Austin, had three children, and raised a family. That was a full-time job, especially since I homeschooled the kids until they were about nine years old. I never thought much of public education in Texas, especially in the boonies. Those Texas kids can't even speak proper English. The teachers can hardly speak good English, certainly not like the English my father taught me. When Daddy gave his sermons, his English was perfect. He was a teacher for the whole community. Anyway, after my last child finished fourth grade, all three kids were in a private school in Austin. Then I suddenly had more time. Of course, my husband was always busy at the ranch, but I didn't like ranch life too much. We got a small condo in Austin, which is where I wanted to be. And so, we lived apart during the week, and on weekends, I would go to the ranch or he would come to Austin. It worked out great. I could be near a library and take courses and be with people who were like-minded, instead of being isolated on the ranch. Then I got the idea that I should finally finish my education and get my college degree. That's when I realized that I'd better hurry up because I could come down with macular degeneration, like my daddy. So here I am. Tell me about my drusen. Do I have time to do two more years of college?"

As she was talking, her gray ponytail wagging from side to side during her agitated speech, I started the eye exam. Her vision was 20/20 in both eyes, and there were no abnormalities except for very mild cataractous opacities of both lenses and drusen of the macula.

"You do have drusen in both eyes. As you probably know, having done your research, these are small deposits under the central retina. They are made up of the by-products of the very rapid metabolism of the retina and are usually gobbled up by the pigment epithelial cells, just under the retina. These cells are the local garbage collectors, but in some older folks, this collection system does not work well and debris accumulates. Hence, drusen."

"Sounds like retinal poop to me." She chuckled. "You need to find a better way to let the retina do its business. A retina laxative is what I need." She was laughing.

"It's sort of interesting what you say. We and a few other institutions have been looking at that. It seems that—and we are not sure yet—some vitamins, like A and C, as well as zinc, may actually help clear up the poop or, at least, slow down its accumulation. We'll probably find out pretty soon if these vitamins work."

"I hope you do, and of course, let me know as soon as *you* know."

"Absolutely."

We then continued our discussion for another twenty minutes. It was obvious that she wanted to learn more about the retina and the pigment epithelium than I could ever teach her in a short time, so I suggested that she go to the internet and search for *drusen*.

"I don't think you'll find it under *retinal poop*!" "I'll do it, and then we'll talk some more."

When she left, she had an appointment for six months later. I had told her that we could check her twice a year for the foreseeable future, until her drusen started to change.

The next two visits were very similar. The exam was unchanged, and we did a lot of talking. She had learned a great deal about macular degeneration and drusen and wanted to know the latest findings in our research. She had started taking a citrus bioflavonoid pill recommended by a health food store and wanted to make sure that there was nothing damaging in the formula. She was yearning to enroll at the University of Texas to take courses to complete her undergraduate degree. She was waiting for her acceptance letter. It made her slightly nervous that she had heard nothing for several months, because she had noticed that she seemed to need more light to see clearly. I assured her that it was not macular degeneration but rather the early cataracts.

"Just about everybody experiences that after sixty or seventy, when cataracts start," I told her.

"Well, all my seventy-watt light bulbs are now a hundred watts."

Six months later, the drusen deposits had increased, and some had coalesced, especially in one eye. We again took photographs, as we had done before, to document the change. Her vision in one eye had also worsened slightly. We talked about the change, which had been gradual. I told her about dry and wet degeneration and that the latter could produce a sudden change. If that happened, she should call right away, because that would be due to a subretinal vascular leak, which could be sealed with a laser. Meanwhile she should continue her vitamin pill.

"And I'm also taking these eye drops which the health store recommended. It seems to increase contrast and makes it easier to read. I need that now because I'm a student again at UT, majoring in English."

Not recognizing the name on the bottle, I read the label, which listed a number of vitamins which, as far as I knew, were not pharmacologically active in the eye.

"I really have to get that degree so I don't let my father down. He was always pushing me to go back to school and become an English professor . . . and a poet. I used to write poetry when I was a kid and then again at college. Several times, when I helped Daddy with his sermons, he used one of my short poems—they were four lines long—as part of the sermon. At Bryn Mawr, I took two poetry classes. Now I am taking another one. We are reading

Paradise Lost by John Milton. It's fantastic, so eloquent! Milton was a very educated man, had travelled a lot, and spoke several languages, including Latin. I know that I'll never write as well as he did, but I need more education to come even close."

"I'm sure you know that Milton went blind later in his life."

"Oh, yes, and he wrote a poem about it."

She hesitated for a moment.

"It starts like this, 'When I consider how my life is spent ere half my days in this dark world and wide,' and then he asks the question, which I also ask myself, 'Does God exact day labor, light denied?' My answer to that question is yes, an unequivocal yes. My own father expected something of me, more than being a ranch wife, and I suppose my other father, the one in heaven, also does."

"That's very philosophical. I guess nothing will stop you, not even some vision problems. But let's make sure that you, unlike Milton, never go blind. I think we have some tools today that were not available then." For a moment, I thought of the poem and remembered how it ended. "But you know the last line of that poem, don't you?" It is 'They also serve who only stand and wait.'

"But that's not my style, and it wasn't Milton's either. He continued to write almost to his death. I think his wife helped him put it on paper."

"From what I remember, historians believe that he probably had glaucoma, so he may have had a small piece of central vision left until the end, although all his side vision was gone, making it dark. That would explain the words *dark world* and also help us understand that he was still able to do some writing until he died."

For a few moments, we said nothing, thinking about our conversation. Then she started again.

"I don't want to sound presumptuous or arrogant, but Milton and I have a lot in common. The more I learn about him in class, the closer I feel. It's uncanny! We both had a strong religious background and fathers who insisted on the best education, including private tutors and special schools. We both valued our personal freedoms and made special arrangements with our spouses so that we could be alone some of the time. We both wrote poetry. And now, this business with vision problems. Amazing. I can really identify with him."

During the next couple of years, Sally's macular degeneration worsened. Although it was dry and slowly progressive at first, it became wet with multiple episodes of vascular leaks in both eyes. She was now taking a special multivitamin with zinc and lutein, which had been shown to slow the progression of the disease. I performed multiple laser treatments to seal the leaks, as she continued to lose some vision. Before reading became really difficult, she was able to get her BA degree in English, a copy of which she faxed me. She started to work for her master's degree, but reading became more difficult all the time, slowing her progress. She used books on tape daily and even had her daughter put some textbooks on tape. When she used glasses or magnifiers, they never seemed to do the job. Although she must have been frustrated, she never lost her curiosity and zest for life. She and I had long conversations about eye research, which gave her hope that some breakthrough would happen soon, which might cure her.

One day, when she was scheduled for another eye exam, she did not show up. I called her at home and left a message. A few days later, I called her daughter, who had been driving Sally to her appointments for over a year. She explained that her mother had just been diagnosed with pancreatic cancer. She had been feeling badly but had now developed severe stomach and back pain. She refused painkillers because she wanted to be mentally clear enough to write poetry. She underwent a celiac plexus injection to mitigate the pain.

During the last few months of her life, I spoke to her several times. Her attitude remained positive, as did her interest in eye research. She still wanted to know every detail about what was going on in our department and elsewhere.

A few months after she died, her daughter called. She also wanted to know what research was going on and stated that she wanted to stay in touch with us. I told her that in June, there would be a big graduation party for our residents, which would be attended by everyone in the department, including all the researchers and many local ophthalmologists from San Antonio and also Austin. I told her that we would invite her.

After the invitations had gone out, she called to ask if it might be appropriate for her to say something at the graduation dinner. She wanted to congratulate the residents on their choice of profession and tell some of her mother's story about the importance of the ophthalmologist in a person's life. Naturally, I agreed to her request.

At the party, a number of speeches were given. Hers turned out to be almost like a fundraising speech. She told her mother's story and even read a small poem, which Sally had written recently. It talked about eyesight and insight, that you could lose one without the other. Then she talked about eye research and how it had postponed Sally's blindness and permitted her to obtain her BA degree. It had also always kept up her hopes for a cure. She encouraged the audience always to support medical research, even if they did not participate in research themselves.

To the residents, she said, "Even if you are just a practicing eye doctor, you can always make a research donation, especially to your alma mater."

At the end of the speech, she asked me to come to the podium, where she handed me a check for $250,000.

"I hope this can start a research endowment."

Chapter 2

IRON LADY

She had cleverly developed a friendly relationship with someone in the dean's office at the medical school so that she would always know when a new faculty member or dean was being hired. As head and owner of Mi Casa, one of the largest real estate companies in town, this was a very useful way to obtain new clients, especially those who would be able afford a more expensive house. Although she and her husband had lived in San Antonio for more than thirty-five years, she had remained an Easterner at heart, from Upstate New York, and had graduated summa cum laude from Mount Holyoke College in Massachusetts. There, she was voted most likely to succeed. During college, she had met Joe, a Yale student majoring in geology, and shortly after their graduations, they married, had two children, and moved to Tampico in Tamaulipas, Mexico, bordering Texas. Joe was a consultant to companies that made parts for oil drilling, and Nancy was busy learning Spanish and bringing up the children. After six years, to take advantage of American schools, they moved to San Antonio, where she opened a real estate office. Being bilingual herself by now, the business grew quickly, and after a few years, she commanded a group of more than a dozen English-and Spanish-speaking agents.

THE EYE: WINDOW TO BODY AND SOUL

When I arrived in San Antonio, having been recruited to become chairman of ophthalmology at the University of Texas medical school, I was told that Nancy Oppenheim might call us, which she did the day after we arrived. She had done her homework and knew that we were temporarily renting and would be looking for a piano teacher for our oldest son, and so we ended up with a piano teacher even before we bought a house.

During the next couple of months, Nancy took us all around town and gave us a great education about different neighborhoods. Her background in the Northeast made communication easy, and we soon became friends. She understood my desire to build a truly academic department, for which I would need the support of the community, and also realized that living close to other academicians and professionals would be productive for my job and most comfortable for the whole family. Within two months, she found us a small house in one of the best, and historic, neighborhoods, where many of the old San Antonio families lived. There was enough land around the house to permit expansion, which we accomplished in short order.

Over the next couple of years, we saw Nancy and Joe, frequently reminiscing, among other things, about Yale and Mount Holyoke and how many times we must have driven that road between them, which we all remembered fondly. Then, Nancy developed some visual symptoms. She called me at home about blurry vision. At first it seemed like it was bilateral, but then, when she covered one eye and then the other, she realized that it was only in her right eye. By now, she was seventy-two years old, the perfect age for macular degeneration. I saw her the next day, performed the exam, which did show some swelling in the right central retina (macula) and tiny hemorrhages. Angiography demonstrated a leak under the retina near the center, as I had suspected. Her vision was 20/70, so she could still see some of the larger letters on the chart. Today, we would treat such leaks with intraocular injections of an antineovascular drug, but then, in 1984, we only had the laser to seal the leaks. The problem with that treatment, however, was that the laser caused a burn, a small retinal scar, which would destroy vision wherever the burn was placed. Thus, central burns would lead to permanent central vision loss. Burns next to the center would produce small blind spots next to whatever the patient would look at, which was definitely noticed by the patient but could be tolerated, especially if it was only in one eye. In fact, a paracentral scar was sometimes not even noticed by some patients. So it was with Nancy after her laser treatment. She was not one to complain anyway, but she insisted that the scar did not bother her. Her vision improved.

During the next year, I had to repeat the laser treatment several times but ultimately could not contain the relentless progress of the disease, leaving her with a scarred macula and 20/200 vision, equivalent to the big E on the chart. Both she and I became well aware that destructive surgical approaches to macular degeneration would never be the answer and that a medical treatment would eventually be needed. That turned out to take another twenty-five years to be discovered.

A few months later, she developed symptoms in her left eye. Again, the same scenario occurred. At first, there was containment of the process with visual recovery, but then recurrences were frequent. This time, I became more aggressive with the laser. With leaks all around the very center of the macula, I treated within millimeters of the center in a letter C pattern, leaving the very center as well as an opening on the temporal side untreated. Later, she would describe to me that the blind spot from the scarring was like a large black whale with its mouth open, through which she could see. Because I did not dare to treat more, the residual leakage did diminish her vision to 20/70, but there it remained. This meant that, because her peripheral vision was excellent, permitting her to navigate, she was now legally blind and could not drive a car anymore. Furthermore, she could only read with a magnifying glass—a slow process.

As a legally blind person in Texas, she took advantage of all the benefits available through the State and the local office of the nonprofit national organization Prevent Blindness America. She obtained an additional deduction on her federal income tax; obtained a collection of magnifiers, some equipped with a light; rented a large desktop magnifier for documents; arranged the ability to call information on the telephone without being charged so she would not have to read the phonebook's small print; and bought a talking wristwatch to tell her the time of day. She also carried a golf ball in her pocketbook, which she placed on the floor of houses to be sold to see whether or not the building was level. She convinced Joe to drive her wherever she needed to go and thus was able to continue her real estate work. Amazingly, most of her agents never realized how limited her vision was.

Then, Joe had a small stroke and another massive one a few days later, which killed him. My wife and I helped with the funeral arrangements, which were quickly completed under the direction of Nancy's daughter. She was now alone at home.

A few days later, we managed to convince Nancy to get a driver. Being in San Antonio, there were always Mexican immigrants who were looking for part-time work, and we quickly found Enrique Palmez, a polite, formal, gentlemanly, and very appreciative sixty-five-year-old American immigrant, who had been born and raised in Mexico and worked part-time as a hearse driver for a funeral home. He even owned a chauffeur uniform and cap. Since his other work was sporadic, Mr. Palmez was available almost any time Nancy needed him. An arrangement was made to let Enrique take Nancy's car home and use it to drive to appointments. We all thought that would be best since it would make it impossible for her, at the spur of any moment, to drive somewhere by herself, which would be dangerous.

During those days, I spoke to Nancy frequently, and my wife even took her to lunch. She seemed to adjust pretty well to her new situation and told me about her daily routine of taking an early morning swim in the pool of her condominium, after which she would be picked up by Enrique to take her to the office. There she would be for at least three hours. The afternoon was for seeing new houses and occasionally having an open house for potential buyers. However, there were, in her conversation, occasional hints of despondence. I suggested that she see her general doctor and called him to recommend some sort of antianxiety or antidepression medication, which he prescribed. I also saw her in my office to make certain that more visual loss was not occurring.

As she was sitting opposite of me in the exam chair and exchanging pleasantries, I asked her what the medication was which her internist had prescribed.

"I don't know the name of it, but here, I'll show you the bottle." She opened her pocketbook to search for the container. I looked down to help her find it when I saw the gun, a small ivory-handled revolver.

"What the heck is that, Nancy? You have a gun? Is it loaded?"

She looked up sheepishly as she shoved it to me, fully loaded with nine bullets.

"You know, many of my agents have guns to protect themselves when they have an open house. You never know who's going to come in."

"But have you always had a gun?"

"No, I just bought it."

"Nancy, tell me truly, did you just buy that because you were depressed?" I was now holding her hand. She did not answer, and as she looked up at me, a tear rolled down her cheek.

"I just don't think you need a gun. I don't think that this lovely hand of yours was ever meant to pull a trigger. If you have an open house or are meeting a client, why don't you just have Enrique stay with you? He drops you off anyway. And leave that gun at the office or get rid of it completely. I care too much for you to have you have an accident with it."

She blinked before she answered, "Thanks for the lecture," then she smiled.

Later, I called her daughter, who said that she also would try to convince her mother to keep Enrique around during meetings with clients. A few weeks later, when I spoke to Nancy again on the telephone, I casually asked her where the gun was now.

"At the office, in my desk, just like you told me to do."

THE EYE: WINDOW TO BODY AND SOUL

As the weeks went by, Nancy's vision remained stable, and she would mention how glad she was that the whale continued to have his mouth open. "If he ever closes his mouth, I'd really be blind."

It may have been a couple of years later—she was now in her late seventies—that Nancy developed other symptoms, which she thought were visual. She wasn't sure whether it was really double vision or not. Certainly, it made her dizzy, and she would have to sit down to let it pass. At times, it just took a few minutes, but at other times, it might take hours for the dizziness to go away. "If I stay standing, I'm afraid that I might fall," she informed me. I saw her again in the office. I could not elicit any double vision, and her acuity was still 20/70 in the left eye. I listened to her carotid arteries with my stethoscope on both sides of her neck, but there was no sound to indicate blockage, and I could feel a good carotid pulse on both sides. Still, I thought that there might be a vascular explanation for her symptoms.

"The next time that you have these symptoms, let Enrique bring you to the office."

A few weeks later, she showed up with Enrique, who was pushing her in a wheelchair, which he had found near the front door of the building. I immediately brought her into an exam room, repeated a cursory eye exam, which showed no change. She really did not have double vision but seemed somewhat disoriented. Before I listened to her carotid arteries again, I took her hand and felt for her pulse. It was at first hard to feel the pulse in her wrist, but then it was obvious that she was having an episode of atrial fibrillation—a very irregular pulse, the typical irregular irregularity, not just an occasional dropped heartbeat.

I took the blood pressure, which was 82/40—dangerously low. This was clearly a problem and most likely the cause of her dizziness.

Immediately, I called the Cardiology Department, and one of the nurses came down to pick her up and to get her seen right away. She was admitted to the hospital and stayed for two days, during which they put her on blood thinners and also found that the drug quinidine could regulate her heartbeat. After she went home, she felt much better, and her double vision, or dizziness, disappeared and did not recur. Her vision also remained stable, and she continued to run her realty business, until her death at age eighty-nine. There had been no way to stop her from working till the very end.

Before she died and was at our house for cocktails, she did say something that I continue to remember verbatim, "Wick, you really have done a lot for me. First, you saved my eyesight so that I could continue to work. Then you saved my life . . . twice, once with the gun and then again with the atrial fibrillation. Thanks."

Chapter 3

Elite

By the time I saw Howard as a patient, he was already in his late seventies and a well-known prominent member of the city's aristocracy, whom I had been fortunate to meet on several previous occasions, mostly related to fundraising for the art museum. He was an unmarried Southern gentleman, who traced his American ancestry back to the Civil War, in which a forefather on his mother's side played a prominent role as a general under Robert E. Lee. Another distant family member was Woodrow Wilson. These family ties undoubtedly contributed to his fascination with military confrontations, particularly during World War I, details of which he had studied exhaustively. He even had a war room in his house, where multiple large tables were set up depicting various military maneuvers, using hundreds of hand-painted lead soldiers to illustrate military positions and strategy of famous battles. Every year, Howard gave a fundraising party at his house, which offered him the opportunity to expound on the reasons for success or failure in battle—whether it was Ypres, Verdun, or somewhere else. I and the other attendees learned a lot of history on those occasions and also got a dose of philosophy about man's seemingly incessant need to wage war.

Howard's much younger friend, an Episcopal clergyman and confidant of the wealthy, had telephoned me days before about Howard's eye problem. It had started two weeks ago, just a few days after Howard had returned from Europe. As I was later told, he had first gone to Moscow and St. Petersburg, where he had two wealthy clients of the new Russian ruling class, whom he advised about their international investments. Then, as usual, to nurture his hobby of antique collecting, he had visited London and then Paris, where he could mix business with pleasure, since several other clients of his small but select investment advisory firm lived on the outskirts of those cities. He had bought some small bronze pieces, one was a bust of Wellington, and had shipped them to the United States. Then, he had boarded the night train to Geneva, which was always his last stop in Europe. There, he had a routine. He checked into the Richemond Hotel, always in the same room overlooking the lake and the Jet d'Eau from the tall windows in the third-floor. This was where he could relax better than anywhere. He had to explain nothing to anyone. The doorman greeted him by name and automatically took his suitcase to his room. The registration desk had his key ready in an envelope. There were no papers to sign. The window table in his room had fresh flowers, and the mini bar had champagne and Laphroaig single-malt scotch, his favorite. Because he had stopped in the lobby for a few minutes, scanning the front pages of the *Manchester Guardian*, the *London Times*, and the *International Herald Tribune*, he found his bag already unpacked—with his suits, shirts, and ties neatly hanging and his underwear and socks properly arranged in the top two drawers of the dresser. His shoes had been polished.

Having arrived in the early morning, well rested after being rocked to sleep by the cadence of the train's wheels on the track as he lay down in the comfortable private sleeper compartment, he was ready for his customary schedule. After a prolonged breakfast with brioches, two soft-boiled eggs, ham, and marmalade, accompanied by a large pot of tea, he spent more than an hour reading various international newspapers. Then, he took a long walk—first across the street past the many flowerbeds, then along the water's edge, where tourists were already beginning to line up for the sightseeing boat trips. He then crossed the end of the lake on the first bridge to a highly manicured garden in front of a row of five-story buildings, housing shops, restaurants, and hotels. Looking up to the top of one of them, he saw the familiar huge illuminated sign for Harry Winston, his friend, advertising elite jewelry and watches. He would probably see Harry later. He always came to the bar at the Richemond around five o'clock.

Howard walked through the gardens along the lakefront, close to the Jet D'Eau fountain, and sat down on a bench in the sun. Across the water, he could see his hotel. He loved this unique spot on earth. Mothers with children passed by. Older couples walked slowly, some with canes like he himself had. The city was bustling with people talking and laughing, trolleys and automobiles competed for noisy dominance, pigeons fluttered about, and an occasional seagull swooped by—or was it some other bird?—this far from the sea. He could smell a bakery and coffee.

Around 11:30 AM, he walked back to the hotel, retracing his steps, taking a good half hour to do so, pausing several minutes to watch the schools of fish in the rapids under the bridge. He could have done it much faster, but there was no reason to hurry. He certainly did not need his cane for this short walk, but it gave him comfort and provided some stability when his feet had to negotiate the occasional stretch of cobblestones. Moreover, he was very proud of his cane, a black shellacked stick with an ornately carved solid-gold handle. The inscription read: "To Woodrow Wilson, from his great friend, David Lloyd—George."

Lunch was in the breakfast room of the hotel, a shrimp quiche with white wine. Then came the nap. He needed that to get ready for his massage. For years, he had used a Thai masseuse, Achara, who had been recommended by the hotel. Originally, she had been brought to Geneva by the previous French ambassador to Thailand, where she was hired to do a variety of chores in the ambassador's residence. She had quickly become an invaluable aide to the ambassador's wife, giving advice about Thai food in the kitchen and Thai social customs and protocol—particularly useful for dinner parties. The ambassador himself also learned to appreciate her talents as a masseuse, specializing in Asian deep-tissue massage, an unexpected expertise from a woman who had originally been hired as a maid and cleaning lady. When the ambassador was reassigned to Geneva to be the permanent representative of France to the European headquarters of the United Nations, he had brought Achara along. As time passed, she had, with the help of the ambassador's recommendation, developed a small private massage business, at first serving his friends but later, as her word-by-mouth reputation grew, expanding her clientele to several dozen foreign nationals in finance, banking, and government. This was how Howard had met her, so every year, when he was in town, she would come to the hotel and cater to his pleasures.

When he awoke from his nap, there was a red blinking message on his telephone. It was from Achara, telling him that she had a bad cold. However, her daughter Areva could come. She had been in Geneva more than a year, escaping from a bad marriage in Thailand, and had been helping her mother almost daily. The message further said, "She is just as good as I am and a lot stronger. She'll be waiting in the lobby at half past three."

When Areva came to the room, having been sent by the concierge, Howard could see the family resemblance to her mother. She was young and beautiful, with long burned-sienna hair, brown eyes, full lips, bronze skin, and moved like a graceful dancer. The massage routine was similar to what he had experienced before and, if anything, was more extensive and thorough. He was completely satisfied and exhausted when she finished.

That evening, he had dinner with Janice Evins, the wife of a longtime friend, also in the investment management business, who was away for a few days seeing clients in Riyadh. She had driven in from Nyon, not far away on the shore of Lake Geneva, and had given him the satisfying opportunity to be seen with a glamorous woman for whom he could play the role of a perfect, gracious host.

The next day, he repeated his routine and even asked Areva to return for another session. That evening, he ran into Harry Winston at the Richemond bar, and the two old friends had dinner together in the formal hotel dining room. On the following day, Howard, using his favorite airline, Swissair, returned to the United States.

Two days later, one eye began to bother him. He called his friend Father Martin, who came over and took him to see Arthur Pierce, Howard's private internist, who immediately prescribed gentamycin eye drops—four times a day in the right eye—and warned him that should the discomfort and redness become bilateral, he could use the drops in both eyes. In another two days, the problem, although it remained in one eye only, was no better. The eye looked red and weepy and felt swollen and slightly painful. Howard carried a small box of Kleenex with him around the house to wipe the discharge from his eye. He cancelled his appointments. Any business he had to do was done over the telephone. Arthur Pierce suggested that he see an optometrist, whose office was in the same building. The optometrist assured him that the eye itself was not involved and that this just represented a bad conjunctivitis. After checking in a reference booklet, which was lying on his desk, he suggested that Dr. Pierce prescribe an additional different class of antibiotic eye drop, Cefazolin, also to be taken four times daily. "That should take care of it."

During the next few days, Dr. Pierce visited his friend Howard at his home almost daily. He considered himself an old-fashioned doctor from the good old days, who still made house calls regularly for his small but elite patient clientele. The conjunctivitis did not improve, even when he changed the medication frequency to six times daily. The purulent drainage continued to be profuse, and Howard was continually cleaning his face with a tissue. At times, he had to use a wet washcloth, because the pus had dried and caked on his cheek.

Another appointment to the optometrist again confirmed that the inside of the eye was not involved and that the combination of an aminoglycoside and a cephalosporin, both broad-spectrum antibiotics, should cure the problem.

When Father Martin called me and told me the story of the relentless conjunctivitis, I decided to see Howard the same afternoon.

Knowing how irritable this impatient man would be in a crowded waiting room, I scheduled him for 5:00 PM, when most of the patients, as well as the staff, would have left already. Only one desk clerk and one technician were still in the office when he arrived. I watched him slowly traverse the waiting room with his cane, looking down at the floor to make sure there were no obstacles. I immediately escorted him to an exam room and started with the preliminary testing, while the tech watched. Since I had already heard the detailed history from Father Martin over the telephone, my conversation was limited.

At first, the most striking observation was the large amount of yellow-green pus dripping from his eye. His lids and lashes were covered with it, as was the Kleenex tissue with which he was repeatedly wiping his cheek.

I put on some rubber gloves, wiped much of the pus on his eyelids away, and was able to test his vision, after Howard blinked away the residue. It was excellent. The pupils were small but equal. Eye movements were normal but caused slight pain. There was no sign of intraocular inflammation, but the peripheral cornea, after I had irrigated the remaining pus away, did show surface irregularities and some small white spots, so-called stromal infiltrates. I told Howard that the infection was beginning to attack the eye itself and that it was time to find exactly what the organism was that caused the pus. In my mind, I reviewed the story of Howard's trip and wondered what else I had missed. Could this be gonorrhea? Almost nothing else could cause that much yellow discharge. What else had he done in those two weeks that I did not hear about?

With a sterile cotton-tipped applicator, I smeared some of the pus onto several agar plates, which were always kept in our refrigerator, and also streaked the thick yellow material onto several glass slides to form a thin layer for staining purposes. The tech took them down to the hospital laboratory immediately. The culture results would be available in two days, but the stains would be done within the hour.

I let the tech and the receptionist go home and completed the patient chart, while Howard waited silently. Then, we had a chance to talk.

THE EYE: WINDOW TO BODY AND SOUL

"Howard, can you think of anything that might have caused this infection? Were you around other people who had the same thing? Were you near any animals—dogs, cats—that you played with or touched? How about children? And what about that Thai girl who gave you the massage? Was she clean?"

"Oh my heavens, yes" was his immediate response. "She was wonderful and . . . beautiful," he said slowly and emphatically. He smiled impishly as he spoke and, for a moment, must have tightened his scalp muscles so that many of his facial and brow wrinkles flattened and disappeared, giving him a sudden youthful appearance. Although the change was fleeting, I could see how he must have looked as a much younger man.

"Tell me about her," I asked. "What all did you do?"

"Well, she does this deep massage, pushing and pulling on everything. Then she has me lie on my stomach and sits on—like, she straddles my lower back and pulls my shoulders up. She must be very strong, although she doesn't look it. It really stretches my back and loosens me up, although it hurts when she does it. Then, she kneads every back muscle from top to bottom. And then she does the same things on my front."

As I listened to him, I began to wonder if this sensual experience had resulted in sex, especially since he was so enthusiastic about telling me the details.

"So what were you wearing?" I asked. "Oh, just a towel."

"And what about her?"

"She had on one of those short bathrobes, you know, like you might see in a Japanese bathhouse—very professional!"

I was coming to the conclusion that indeed the massage had been more intimate than I had originally suspected, but I asked no more questions about it. I closed the conversation with the comment: "Sounds like it was great." He nodded and smiled.

I excused myself to look for the pathology smear results, which came in another twenty minutes, and showed the unequivocal presence of gram-negative diplococci, which could only be gonorrhea. There was no need to wait for the cultures to prove it. That would delay the treatment, which should be started immediately to prevent the cornea from being involved more. Corneal ulcers could certainly lead to perforations, which might even cause loss of the eye.

I told Howard that he might have gotten the infection from his massage therapist but did not mention the word *gonorrhea*. I think that he understood.

Treatment was started immediately, as the hospital pharmacy next door was able to formulate a strong penicillin eye drop to be used hourly. I showed Howard how to administer the drops himself so as not to contaminate other people, like his housemaid, who might have been recruited to perform this duty. We also discussed hygiene such as Lysol spray, frequent handwashing, and limiting his social contacts. During the next hour, I kept Howard in the office and watched him using the eye drops.

Meanwhile, I called Dr. Pierce to share the story. He then prescribed the systemic antibiotics also needed to control the infection, starting with an intramuscular dose of ceftriaxone, followed by several weeks of oral antibiotics. Both Arthur Pierce and I saw Howard almost daily following this evening. The conjunctivitis improved rapidly without further complications, and no other sign of gonorrhea was found.

Later, Arthur Pierce, during one of his frequent discussions with me, wondered if Howard might ever have had any other venereal disease. Although there was no specific reason to suspect this, the gonorrheal conjunctivitis had made him think. He asked me if I had ever tested Howard for syphilis. My negative response promoted him to say, "Well, maybe we should. It can't hurt."

And so blood was drawn and submitted for two different syphilis tests, one a nonspecific (VDRL) and the other a more specific, the FTA-ABS. Pierce called me about the results: the first was negative, but the second was positive. He then did a spinal tap, the results of which were equivocal. Pierce then decided to treat for chronic syphilis, even though no systemic symptoms were present. A course of high-dose penicillin was started.

Several months later, when I saw Howard again during routine follow-up, I performed a thorough and complete examination, including a dilated peripheral retinal exam. I noticed considerable pigmentation in and under the retina, which I had previously noted several years before but ascribed to aging. However, now that I knew about the positive blood test, I recognized that the pigment was not diffuse in the periphery of the retina but rather more localized in three distinct patches—typical of past inflammation, so-called chorioretinitis. I mentioned it to Arthur Pierce. Was this evidence of an old syphilitic inflammation, which might have occurred many years ago? This unanswered question also made me wonder if Howard's frequent use of his beautiful cane, which he liked to show off to everyone, was really a needed support to hide a walking disability, the result of chronic syphilis. I was glad that Pierce had decided to treat Howard. It seemed the right thing to do.

Part VIII

Divine Intervention

Chapter 1: Salvation 205
Chapter 2: The Power of the Church 212
Chapter 3: Oops 220

Chapter 1

SALVATION

The story was typical. He had suddenly developed the sensation of flashing lights on his right side. He noticed it at dusk, when he was getting his dinner ready. Then, the next morning he saw dozens of black spots, which he quickly figured out were from his right eye. They bothered him as he tried to read. Then, by lunchtime, he lost some vision. It was like a curtain was being pulled across his eye, from below upward. He called his eye doctor, who recognized the symptoms of a retinal detachment and, without even seeing him, referred him directly to our retina office.

When Sam Rothblum arrived, he was not happy. He asked the receptionist how many minutes he would have to wait before someone would call his name. He corrected her pronunciation.

"It is pronounced *Rotebloom*. Everybody always screws it up. Why can't they say it right? Are they uneducated?"

He sat down, fidgeting with a magazine and repeatedly checking his vision by covering one eye with his hand and then the other. After ten minutes, the tech called him. She had already been told how to pronounce his name. It surprised him, and he cracked a faint smile as he rose to follow her.

The tech's exam and mine showed no surprises. The retina in the right eye was torn in three places, which had caused a detached retina with some bleeding. I explained that the retina, which normally is the inner lining in the back of the eye, had gotten some fluid under it so that it was ballooned forward, away from its blood supply, and also not flat, so no good images could be formed on it.

"It's like trying to take a picture with a camera when the film is all folded and crumpled." I think he understood.

"Repairing detached retinas is what we do a lot of. In your case, we should probably do this soon, in a day or so. The results are pretty good—about 85 percent or more chance of success."

"What if it doesn't work?" "Then we'll try again."

I then asked him some other questions about his home situation to find out how much support he would need following the operation.

"And by the way, you seem to have a slight accent. Is it New York Yiddish or what? It sounds quite German to me."

"You're right, it's German, but I've lost most of it. I've been here more than twenty years."

He then proceeded to tell me a long story about his amazing life. He was brought up near Hamburg and was seventeen when World War II broke out. The Nazis had already invaded Poland, and anti-Semitism was on the rise. His parents didn't know what to do. Should they just flee and leave everything behind? His father ran a successful grocery store and did not want to give that up. His mother was more inclined to escape through Holland or Denmark. The procrastination doomed all action. They stayed in Hamburg, and then, in May 1940, Germany invaded Holland. All Jews were quickly identified, and many, within weeks, were transported by truck and train eastward to concentration camps in Poland. The Rothblum family was included.

When they got to the camp, they were immediately divided into groups by sex and age. Because Sam looked older than his seventeen years, he was put with adult males, the same as his father. The process was very militaristic, with officers shouting commands and heels clicking, but there was something incongruous happening at the same time: he heard music. It must have been a string quartet playing somewhere. He recognized it. It was a string quartet by

Mozart, which he had played himself on the cello as part of a group in Hamburg.

"I can play on that cello," he told a guard who was pushing him in line. "Do you have an orchestra here?"

The guard stopped pushing.

"Yes, of course, and a very good one" was the proud answer.

"How can I get to play in the orchestra?"

"How do I know you can play?" "That's what I do. I play music."

"And he is a great cellist," his father stated pompously.

"Come with me," said the officer, as he grabbed him by the sleeve. That was the last time he saw his father.

During the next four years, Sam played in the camp orchestra and, together with the other musicians, was protected from starvation and extermination. The others in his family went to the gas chambers.

"The cello saved my life," he kept saying.

After the war, he made his way back to Hamburg, where he found little solace and finally arranged, through a distant cousin in New York, to come to America in 1948.

"This is so interesting," I said. "That was the same time that *my* family came to the US as well. We went to Connecticut, where my father, also an ophthalmologist, had found a job at Yale University."

"Well, I guess we have something in common. I ended up in Brooklyn."

He then told me that he had met his wife, a second-generation German Jewish girl, in New York, where they both ended up working in a restaurant and got married. Occasionally, he would entertain the restaurant clientele with cello music, accompanied by the owner's wife on the piano.

They lived happily together for over twenty years, until his wife tripped on a subway escalator and fell headfirst down the steps, fracturing her skull. She did not survive.

After that, being alone and wanting to get away from the dangers of the big city, he moved to the Catskills, forty miles north. There he had found a Jewish club with a number of cottages, one of which he bought.

"So now I don't have to go into the city anymore. I can get everything around here, including finding a retinal doctor. And they let me play the cello at the club. We have quite a group of musicians. It's really nice."

Two mornings later, I performed a scleral buckling procedure, at that time the standard of care. During the operation, I noticed some evidence that part of the detached retina inferiorly may have been detached for longer than the two-day history indicated. It included some scarring on the retinal surface, which made it difficult to get the retina back into position. The next day, I told Sam about it, but he wasn't as concerned as I was. A week later the retina was still partially detached, which worsened during the following week. A reoperation was needed!

When we took Sam back to the operating room, it was obvious that the retinal surface scarring was worse. During the three-hour operation, I tried but failed to reattach the retina.

The next morning, my associate and I discussed the problem, and we agreed to follow our usual protocol, which was to let the other surgeon try for the third time. Sam agreed, and another scleral buckling revision was done. It, too, failed.

"Is there anyone who can fix this thing?" Sam wanted to know.

"We can send you to Boston, where our mentor works. Are you willing to go and see him, at least to get a second opinion?"

"Absolutely. He probably didn't teach you guys everything he knows. Maybe I should have gone to him right from the start." He was not joking and was clearly irritated.

As it turned out, the Boston referral was futile. He was told that nothing could be done, but from my point of view, the visit was worthwhile because our mentor had praised our work and given our patient new confidence in us.

During the next couple of years, I saw Sam Rothblum every six months to check his other eye, which never showed any signs of predetachment. Then he called in a panic. The same thing was happening to his remaining good eye. A "curtain" was coming across his vision, and he saw hundreds of red and black spots.

"I'm coming over right now, whether you have time for me or not."

Of course, I saw him within an hour and confirmed the diagnosis of total retinal detachment. His vision was very poor, and he was brought in by a female friend from the club, who led him awkwardly into the exam room. He was terribly upset.

"You have to fix this. We have no choice. *Verdammte Augen*, what can you do? Do I need to go somewhere else? Where can I go? What are my chances? You've got to do better than the last time!"

"Well, we've discussed this before. Our success rate is close to 90 percent, sometimes we have to operate twice to achieve that number, and all the failures are due to that retinal scarring that you had in your other eye. The likelihood of that happening again is very small. We'll get you on tomorrow's schedule." While he listened, his head was down, a picture of despondence.

The next day's surgery went well, but the eye developed preretinal scarring rapidly during the postoperative weeks, creating a recurrence of the detachment. A second operation also failed. Then he went to New York City for a second opinion because "New York always has the best doctors." Unfortunately, a reoperation in the city also failed and left him blind except for the ability to discern light from dark.

Sam's story, however, did not end there. He was able to move from his cottage to an apartment in the main clubhouse, where he found a young aide to help him with daily chores. After a few phone calls, our office enrolled him in a state program to teach him mobility with a white cane and start a Braille program. He learned quickly, being highly motivated, lived in a nurturing environment, had all his meals in the club dining room, and seemed to be doing amazingly well, but he was sad. He stated that he felt lonely in the dark.

During this period, I saw him twice in the office to make sure he was not developing other problems, which sometimes occur in eyes with chronic retinal detachment. On occasion, these problems can lead to constant pain, which, in a blind eye, is a reason for enucleation, the surgical removal of the eye. I certainly would never want to subject him to that procedure.

A few months later, he called and needed to speak to me personally. "I must come and see you again. It is important."

"Why, are you having pain?"

"No, it is something else. When can I come?" I gave him an appointment a week later.

When he arrived, he was accompanied by a pretty middle-aged woman who looked Irish, with white slightly freckled skin and short curly russet hair. She also was visually handicapped, using a white cane, but she obviously could see something, having little problem finding chairs for both of them in the waiting room. I led them to a nearby exam room, where they both sat down in chairs designated for family members. He looked in my direction and smiled, something I had not seen him do for a long time. What made him so different?

"Don't you want to sit in the exam chair?" I asked. He shook his head.

"I don't need an exam. I just need to say a few things." He cleared his throat and took a deep breath.

"Dr. van Heuven, I want to thank you. Had it not been for the fact that you could not fix my stubborn retinas—and I know that you tried very hard—I would never have met my love of loves, this wonderful Margareth." He pointed in her direction.

"The sweetest, most caring woman I have ever met. We were in Braille class together. She made me realize how terrible you must have felt when you failed to fix my eyes. It was bad for me, yes, but also for you. I had never thought of that before. I am sorry that I was such an uncooperative patient. But now, I feel better, much better. I have a love that I never thought could exist. She has helped me move back to my bungalow and, although she is legally blind from macular degeneration, can see just enough to take care of both of us. But the most wonderful happening is that she has gotten me to play the cello again. Practicing the Dotzauer musical ladders is making my fingers more nimble and stronger. I do that every day. Then there are the melodic exercises by Sebastian Lee, which you may not know, but I remember them from the Nazi days. The greatest pleasure, though, is to play the Bach suites for solo cello, which I have never forgotten. And you wouldn't believe it, Margareth has figured out how to accompany me on the piano. She is quite a musician, and although she can't see much, she has a great ear. You know, Dr. van Heuven, this is the second time that the cello has saved my life."

Chapter 2

The Power of the Church

Joe Pernacky's name was well-known in the community. His round and ruddy face was frequently seen on the local TV channel with an aggressive advertisement for his Cadillac dealership, promising to beat anyone else's price by at least five hundred dollars. You would get another one hundred dollars if you had never had a Cadillac before and still another hundred if you traded in your foreign car to buy American. His eighteen-year-old daughter, a pretty, thin-lipped tall blonde, was the model who demonstrated the automobile while he spoke, "If you've never had a Cadillac before, now is the time. It's the best car in the world. You deserve it!" It was an advertisement clearly targeted to the modern American me generation.

I recognized him when he came to the office. He was about five foot ten, weighed about three hundred pounds, and walked with a swagger. He was obviously nervous and had not sat down in the waiting room but instead had paced between the empty chairs. It was before 8:00 AM on a Monday, and the techs were just coming into the office, surprised to see a patient already there. The usual first appointment was not until 8:20 AM.

It was on the day before that his symptoms had started. The weather was miserable—dark, damp, and penetratingly cold—and almost convinced him not to go to church, but he had capitulated

THE EYE: WINDOW TO BODY AND SOUL

and went anyway. He would not let bad weather make him break his Presbyterian routine. He would be a bad example. People expected him to be there. It was good for business to be seen.

The temperature was just below freezing when he stepped onto his driveway. Although there was no new snow, the high humidity of the dark-gray day had formed a shiny thin layer of ice on the asphalt. His feet slid slightly as he opened the car door and got in. The five-minute ride to church was uneventful, but he drove carefully. The morning traffic, although sparse, had helped de-ice the pavement, leaving it wet, good enough for some traction. Once parked, he chose to walk from his car to the church steps through the snow-covered grass on the side of the path, where the crunch of his footsteps assured a firm footing. He felt he was later than usual—with no time for his customary social interactions, which were so important to sustain his stature in the community as a prominent businessman and citizen.

The church was a beautiful example of Jeffersonian architecture, red brick with trim whiter than snow, and six great Doric pillars supporting the ornate frieze. The more-than-a-dozen steps leading up to the three sets of double front doors were flanked by railings and bestowed a commanding presence of the facade on the neighborhood. In his hurry, Joe did not notice the small temporary signs that had been placed near both railings—Watch for Ice, Use Railing. He steamed up the central stair, aiming straight for the open middle doors, slipped, and fell forward, breaking his crash partly with his right elbow but hitting the left side of his face on the next step. His brow and cheekbone bore the brunt of the fall and instantly swelled, but there was no bleeding, and his eye was not hit directly. He scrambled to the side of the steps and put cold snow on his face to stop the edema. After a few minutes, he used the railing to return to his car and went home. On his way into the house, he picked up a little more snow and held it against his face.

Joe's wife was surprised to see him back from church so quickly. She dutifully listened to his story and was clearly glad that he had not hurt himself worse. In fact, the cold snow must have helped, because the redness and swelling of his face was minimal. The greatest damage seemed to be to his psyche. He was angry.

"Damn that church, they should have used salt on the steps." During the next few hours, he perused the Sunday newspaper with all its car dealership ads, had a sandwich with coffee for lunch, and then took a short nap on the couch while the TV showed an ice hockey game. When he awoke, the sky was an even gray, which, combined with the snowy lawn, was glaringly bright, as seen through the large windows of the enclosed winterized porch. He looked to follow a crow, which seemed to dart erratically against the brightness, but whenever he tried to fixate on it, it moved to the left. Then he realized there was no crow, just some large black irregular spot in his vision, not far from the center but moving whenever he moved his eyes. In addition, as he began to pay more attention, he saw dozens of tiny spots, a faint honeycomb of small hair-thin gray connected lines interspersed by tiny perfectly round black dots. All of them moved with eye movement but then slowly came to rest when eye motion ceased. He remembered having a similar experience about a year or so before, during the summer, but that had been less noticeable and disappeared in a few days.

"Could this be from my fall at the church?" he asked his wife.

That night, he called our office. The answering service recommended going to the emergency room, but he insisted.

"Can't you get me in tomorrow morning? I don't want to wait in the emergency room. That will take all night, and then they'll end up just referring me to your office anyway."

The operator, not having the time or interest in an argument, suggested, "Why don't you go to the office early in the morning? They open at eight. Then they can try to fit you in. That's probably the best."

Since I usually arrived at the office early, I had seen him come in at seven fort-five, only minutes after the office manager had unlocked the front door. When the first tech arrived, I told her to get the patient ready so I could see him before our regular schedule started.

When she brought him into my exam room, she had already done an abbreviated medical history and checked the vision and the eye pressure. He could see 20/20 in his right eye but only 20/40 in his left eye. Pressures were normal. His left cheekbone was chafed, slightly red and mildly swollen. Everything else was normal. Suspecting a vitreous detachment, a collapse of the vitreous gel, both eyes were dilated. At first, he objected to the drops in his right eye then acquiesced, after I told him that his right eye, the normal one, was really his only good eye now and therefore was even more important than his left, and I wanted to make sure that at least that eye was normal.

The diagnosis of vitreous detachment and a slight vitreous hemorrhage was confirmed. Interestingly, he also had a vitreous detachment in his good right eye. I explained what a vitreous detachment was, as I demonstrated a large plastic model of an eye to him.

"You see, the eyeball is filled with a clear gel. It fills up the eye and lies against the surface of the retina so that light coming to the eye can be focused by the lens onto the retina in the back, where an image is formed. Now with time, with aging, the vitreous gel slowly begins to liquefy from the center out. And so at your age, your vitreous gel is probably just a balloon, with the wall of the balloon still being gel but the inside of the balloon being all liquid water. Then, and this occurs in almost all older people eventually, the balloon wall gets thinner and thinner, and the balloon finally breaks. It collapses all within the eye, and the water runs out, as the surface of the balloon peels away from the retina. The water then runs up against the retina. As this gel surface peels away from the retina, it may tug on the retina a little bit. Occasionally, it can tear the retina, which is a very thin and fragile layer. If that happens, the gel's water can pass through the tear and start lifting the retina up, away from the next layer of the wall of the eye, where the retina's blood supply is located. The retina is now floating in the middle of the eye, away from its blood supply, and is not flat, like a folded or crumpled film in a camera, unable to take a good picture. That is called a retinal detachment, which is a surgical emergency but can often be repaired. However, even if the vitreous collapses, which we call vitreous detachment and does not tear the retina, like in your case, it almost always pulls a few loose cells away from the surface of the retina. These cells move around with eye motion and cast small shadows onto the retina, which you see as floaters."

"So is that what happened? My gel collapsed?" He was looking up at me from his forward-leaning position in the chair, with his brow raised.

I nodded, but his expression remained incredulous. He seemed insulted.

"What about my retina tearing? Did you take a good look? I sure as hell don't want a retinal detachment. Goddammit, why did I get this? There's nothing else wrong with me. I'm only fifty-seven and in great shape. I'm not some fucking old man. I can lift weights like anybody."

I told him that really it was no big deal and that he had no retinal tear. I was certain. The fact that his vitreous detachment had not done any damage to the retina probably protected him for the rest of his life from ever getting a retinal detachment. In fact, the same was true for his other eye. "You are actually quite lucky," I suggested. "You are much better off than all the people who haven't had their vitreous detachment yet."

Still leaning forward but now facedown, he mumbled to himself, "Those goddamn slippery steps."

When he sat back, he spoke more audibly, "But you know, Doc, these floating things bug the shit out of me. That big floater is right there, right where I want to look. When I look at the paper, it's like a big black bird that prevents me from seeing the letters. Will this go away?"

"Not ever completely, but just like your other eye where you had some black spots before, they will get fewer and smaller, and your brain will actually learn to ignore them."

"Bullshit" was the explosive retort.

I shrugged my shoulders. "You'll see, I promise."

THE EYE: WINDOW TO BODY AND SOUL

"You know, if the church people had only salted the steps, this would never have happened. Maybe I should just sue them."

"C'mon, Joe, don't even think like that." I tried to cajole him, using his first name to personalize the conversation. "This would've happened anyway, church steps or not. Almost everyone who has a vitreous detachment in one eye gets the same thing in the other eye within three years."

"But this happened immediately after I fell. It was definitely caused by the fall."

"Well, it might have happened on that day because you fell, but without your fall, it might have happened a week later or a month or at least this year."

Joe Pernacky left the office, still unhappy. We gave him some disposable sunglasses to combat the outside glare. As he left, he was muttering, "I can't see shit with my eyes dilated like this."

Six weeks later, I saw him again just to make certain that his retina was intact. Now the small hemorrhage had cleared, and my view was optimized. The retina looked fine, and his vision in that eye was 20/20. He was still complaining bitterly about the large central black bird in his vision.

"It really bothers me. I look at a contract, and I really can't see it at all. It's interfering with my work. Sometimes, I think I should quit, but I have all these people working for me, and none of them is capable of running the place. And also, I can't quit. My dealership is the best in the state, and we're making a fortune. If this damn eye forces me to quit, I could never get disability anyway." It was clear he was still very frustrated.

"Give it a little time," I suggested. "You'll be okay."

Several months later, I noticed that the TV ads for his Cadillac dealership had changed. He was no longer the pushy bulldozer star of the ad. Instead, a much younger and slightly awkward young man demonstrated the luxury of the automobile. The following week, the local *Sentinel Observer* had a headline: "PERNACKY SUES CHURCH."

I called Joe and got him to the telephone without difficulty. "Hey, Joe, how are you doing? How's your eye?"

"This goddamn thing is not going away, Doc. It's really screwed up my work. I can't stand it!"

"I noticed your name in the paper. Are you really suing the church? Is that such a good idea?"

"Well, the church was responsible. If they had taken care of those church steps, this never would have happened. The church has deep pockets. They can handle it."

He then went on to describe how he couldn't read anymore because of this huge floater, which was always in the way. He even suggested that his symptoms were getting worse because the floater was getting larger and affecting his other eye as well. I soon realized that his story was now inconsistent with reality and that he was clearly motivated to make his case seem worse than it was. I had never in my entire career seen or heard of a case of simple vitreous detachment that became intolerable to the point of incapacity. No, in fact, the opposite was usually the case. The patient would see one or more floaters, which were annoying at best, usually located near but slightly to the side of fixation, which would get smaller with time and to which the patient invariably became accustomed.

I asked Joe to come back to see me so that I could check him again, making sure that nothing new was happening in his eyes, such as recurring vitreous hemorrhages, which might occur in diabetes. After all, he was overweight, and judging from his ruddy, round face and short fat neck, as well as the emotional stress he was experiencing, he might now be hypertensive as well. That combination could easily produce retinal vascular problems, which might cause vision problems. However, my examination indicated nothing new. His eye findings were the same, with 20/20 vision bilaterally and evidence of vitreous detachment with a few vitreous floaters. His blood pressure was normal, and his blood glucose test, which I had ordered at a local lab, was also normal.

Six months later, having heard nothing from him or about him, I called him to suggest coming back for another appointment. His wife answered the phone.

"Joe's been real sick lately," she said. "It started with the stomach flu, but he just couldn't get over it. The doctor has given him everything! Then, just the other day, he sent us to a specialist who took a lot of tests, including an MRI. We're just waiting for the results."

I called her back two weeks later. The lab results had been shocking and suggested pancreatic cancer. Several biopsies revealed metastases throughout the body. It was deemed inoperable and too advanced for chemotherapy. Joe was now being given palliative therapy, and hospice was being involved with his care.

The obituary article in the *Sentinel Observer*, three months later, was long and praised Joe Pernacky for his community leadership. He had started as the son of poor Czech immigrant parents and become a successful, wealthy businessman, president of the local chamber of commerce, a pillar of the church, and a generous contributor to the local library. He had succumbed to cancer after a brief illness, with his wife and daughter by his side. Contributions in his memory could be given to hospice or to the Westminster Presbyterian Church.

Chapter 3

Oops

Last year, when I had my first cataract removed, I was astounded at the complex system that was used to prevent operating on the wrong eye. After arriving at the eye clinic and signing in at the outpatient surgery desk, I was taken to the preop area, where I was installed in a special chair, which could be converted into a stretcher/operating table. The nurse asked me, after helping me exchange my shirt for a small gown, which eye was going to be done.

"I hope it's on the chart," I said.

"Yes, it is, but I just want to make sure that your answer matches the chart."

"Well, what does the chart say?"

"I'm not going to tell you until you tell me first."

I guess I was being a difficult patient. Doctors make the worst patients, I had often heard.

"OK, it's the right eye."

She typed it on the computer and then hung a small sign at the foot of the bed. It stated OD (*oculus dexter*), meaning right eye. The next nurse I saw, a few minutes later, introduced herself as an anesthesia assistant. She had a number of questions about recent eye problems and recent medical issues, especially a cold or the flu. She finished by asking which eye was going to be operated.

"It's at the foot of the bed."

"No, I want to hear it from you."

When I told her OD, she also typed it into the computer and then said that my doctor would be right in, before they gave me any sedatives, to talk to me. As she was leaving, he arrived, parting the curtain around my bed. As usual, his voice and manner were full of gravitas, instilling confidence.

"Well, my friend, how is it to be on the receiving end for a change?"

"It's actually quite interesting, although I never did much cataract surgery. My field was retina and melanoma."

"It looks like we're going to do your right eye. That's what my notes say, and that's what you told the nurses. Do you agree?"

I nodded affirmatively. He then proceeded to mark my forehead with a magic marker over my right eye.

"You have quite a system going here. We never did this in retina. Instead, we dilated the eye to be operated and looked in with the indirect ophthalmoscope to see if the dilated eye really had the detachment or the tumor. In retina, that seemed to be the best way to go."

"But that may not be as safe in the case of cataract surgery. Many patients we operate on have some cataract in both eyes, and it is difficult in the OR to tell which eye is worse, especially if you dilate only one. So we still don't know which eye to do first. Instead, we ask the patient."

That day the surgery went well, and my vision improved. However, during the following weeks, my thoughts returned to my preop experience and the last-minute conversation with my surgeon. It reminded me of an episode during one of my first years as an ophthalmologist, when I was a captain in the US Army, stationed at the DeWitt Army Hospital in Fort Belvoir, Virginia.

The fort was located on the Potomac River in Arlington, a few miles north and across the river from Washington, DC. It serviced several military bases, including Fort Belvoir itself, Fort McNair, Quantico Naval Base, and the Pentagon. Across the river, the air force had its own eye clinic at Andrews Air Force Base, and the army had an eye clinic at Walter Reed Army Hospital. The DeWitt eye clinic was busy because of the large number of soldiers it took care of. It was also more interesting than many military base clinics because of the Pentagon, a hub of senior military personnel who were older. Since eye diseases, such as glaucoma and cataract, are more common over the age of forty, we had many patients with those conditions, giving us a more balanced practice as well as a steady surgical volume. The younger soldiers were less interesting, because eye disease is relatively uncommon between ten and forty, except for trauma, allergies, foreign bodies on the eye, and conjunctivitis. Then there were those soldiers who, for whatever reason, were malingering, claiming suddenly not to see out of one or both eyes. What was unexpected, however, was that we saw many children as patients. The joke became that in order to become a staff sergeant, you had to have at least one child with crossed eyes. Indeed, there were many children who were either cross-eyed or walleyed, for a variety of reasons—some congenital, some because they were farsighted around age three, and some because they needed glasses in at least one eye and had never had a vision test. And so, I felt that I needed more training in pediatric ophthalmology and wanted some supervisory assistance to deal with these children. As luck would have it, Marshall Parks, one of the two most famous pediatric ophthalmologists in the US, practiced in Washington and was already accustomed to being a consultant to the military. He agreed to help me, so every month, I would present to him five or six cases, which we would discuss and then decide if eye muscle surgery was indicated and which muscles needed to be recessed or advanced on which eye. It was an unbeatable learning experience and almost turned me into a pediatric ophthalmologist myself.

Then a routine became established. On the second week of every month, I would schedule six muscle operations (strabismus surgery), taking about six hours. It was the same day that the ENT Department, which shared our clinic space with us, also scheduled a similar number of pediatric tonsillectomies, which were very popular in those days, more so than today. We would share one half of the two-room OR, each using a room adjacent to a common workroom, where equipment was sterilized and stored and where we scrubbed our hands before each operation. All cases were done under general anesthesia. While I was scrubbing, the child would be put to sleep. Then the nurse and I would look at the case card, which had the patient's name, the eye to be operated, and the summary of the procedures to be done. This was a critical double check, since each case was different, and once the child was asleep, the eyes often returned to a neutral position, making it impossible to know which eye was the culprit or even whether the child even had strabismus.

One Tuesday, after finishing two cases, I walked into the OR to start the third case. The patient was already asleep. The nurse confirmed that the name was John Thomas and told me it was the right eye, a recession of the lateral rectus muscle. I looked at the patient and noted no sign of strabismus, not unusual. I also noted the child's red hair. I immediately knew that this was not my patient.

"I don't have a patient with red hair!"

"Are you sure?" the nurse asked.

"Absolutely certain."

"But this *is* John Thomas. Look at his armband."

I looked. She was right.

"How can that be?"

At that moment, the circulating nurse ran out of the OR and into the workroom.

"I'll be right back. Wait for me!"

She returned quickly, slightly out of breath.

"You won't believe this. There's a John Thomas on the ENT tonsil list as well. Look at the wristband. Doesn't it say ENT?"

"Yes, it does. This must be *their* patient. But where is *my* patient?"

I was getting concerned.

"Where is he right now?"

"I'll go check," the nurse answered.

She ran out again and came back almost immediately.

"He's in the recovery room. He's just had his tonsils removed!"

No one moved or said anything for a couple of minutes. Then I felt obligated to speak, "Let me just go to the ENT room and speak with them."

As it turned out, the result of the mix-up was better than it could have been. Although the error was clearly the fault of the ENT service, it was their incredible luck that my eye patient was also on the ENT list for a future tonsillectomy, so no harm was done to anyone. It took some deft explaining to the child's parents, but finally they, and we, all took a deep breath, grateful that nothing worse had happened. What I learned was to see every patient personally just before any operation, before they were anesthetized, and use a magic marker somewhere on their face to identify the patient as well as the eye. Thank God for red hair.

As I now look back on the last forty-plus years since that experience, I have heard of many similar errors in ophthalmology and also in other surgical fields, some with devastating effects. Wrong eyes have been operated and sometimes removed. Wrong kidneys have been extirpated, and wrong limbs have been amputated. Thank heaven that we have all learned something from such terrible mistakes. That's why today, we make a patient go through this seemingly redundant system of preop double-and triple-checking, which I had just experienced as a cataract patient.

Part IX

THE OPHTHALMOLOGIST AS A HERO

Chapter 1: She Gave What She Could 227
Chapter 2: Growing Up Fast 233
Chapter 3: I'll Forever Love You..243
Chapter 4: Dependence 251
Chapter 5: Pallbearer..258

Chapter 1

SHE GAVE WHAT SHE COULD

It now seems like such a long time ago, but it was really only sixty years ago that ophthalmologists were beginning to learn what caused diabetics to lose their vision. We knew almost nothing about this vascular change in the retina, and after we learned some of that, it still took many years to develop lasers to treat the vascular problems and stop the bleeding. Then came the recognition that leakage from these sick blood vessels caused an active shrinkage of the vitreous gel, which, as it contracted, pulled the retina—to which it was flimsily attached—forward. This created a retinal detachment, separating the seeing retina away from its blood supply.

I was at the beginning of my academic career and wanted to know more, realizing quickly that collaboration with basic scientists would be necessary to understand what was really happening and why. Having developed an interest in biochemistry during my undergraduate years made me naturally drift toward seeking a biochemical explanation for the clinical changes that were occurring in the eye and causing blindness.

It didn't take long to find Liu Wei Chang, PhD, a Hong Kong–born biochemist who had recently gotten his degree at our university. He had wanted to become a doctor but thought that his English pronunciation was not good enough to communicate with patients, so he thought that biomedical research would be almost as good. We instantly got along and started a collaboration which would last more than forty years. During all that time, there was hardly a workday that I did not see him at least once. It was like a perfect intellectual partnership. I told him about clinical problems and questions I had, and he suggested biochemical experiments that could be done to find answers. At first, he remained employed by his mentor as a postdoc in the Biochemistry Department, but later, after Liu and I got our first NIH grant, he joined our Eye Department full-time. No longer did he have to teach basic biochemistry to medical students, but once a year he still gave a two-hour medical school lecture about biochemistry of the eye.

Our first joint experiment concerned the biochemical analysis of various fluids and tissues in the eye, which, surprisingly, had not been done very much in humans. At first, I was able to obtain samples from the local eye bank, which obtained donor eyes from deceased patients who had signed up to donate their corneas, at their time of death, for the purpose of providing tissue for corneal transplants. The cornea, the transparent front surface of the eye, was the only part of the eye that was used for transplantation. The rest was thrown away. This became a godsend, plentiful and free. As Liu did his analyses, it soon became obvious that specimens varied, which demanded an explanation. The next step, therefore, was to find out more about the donor patient. What was the age, the sex, the medical history? Did the patient have glaucoma, cataract, or some retinal disorder? Could the patient see, and how well?

It took some time to organize, but with the help of the local Lions' Club, which had an interest in eye banking, we were able to get patients to volunteer their pertinent histories at the same time that they signed up for their eye donations.

During the next couple of years, we were able to publish several articles, which basically gave chemical data for human eyes to the research world in order to stimulate other investigators at other institutions to help seek the same answers we were seeking. It was gratifying that several other labs joined in, but the biochemical approach to eye research was not universally appreciated. At one ARVO (Association for Research in Vision and Ophthalmology) meeting in 1971, a well-known physiologist commented publicly that biochemistry of the eye was a waste of time and should never be funded. Fortunately, not everyone agreed.

As our work progressed, we supplemented our source material with fluid samples from living patients who were undergoing cataract, glaucoma, or retina surgery. Again, rather than throw these fluids away during a procedure, we simply collected them in small syringes for analysis. This had never been done before and provided us with considerable new information. At first, we had not considered the need to tell patients that we would be taking samples, but later, we included it in the patient's consent for surgery.

After we had published a few more articles, we summarized our work in lay language, which was published in the Sunday edition of the local paper. We also left copies of it in our patient waiting room and then even sent a copy to every patient in our files, requesting tax-deductible donations for research. By this time, we had two grants, one from Fight for Sight for ten thousand dollars and one from the NIH for eighty thousand dollars. Amazingly, our first letter to patients produced almost another thirty thousand.

Because so many of our patients had diabetes, which was such a common cause of blindness, we especially began to analyze samples from diabetic eyes and compared them to nondiabetics. We specifically wanted to know what made the vitreous gel, which fills up most of the eye and lies up against the retina, shrink and pull away from the retina, causing hemorrhage and retinal detachment. And it was not just shrinkage of the gel. There seemed to be a fibrotic process going on, the formation of scar tissue on the retinal surface, which made the attachment between retina and vitreous much stronger. Then, when the vitreous shrank, it would really pull hard on the retina. What cells were involved in this process? What chemical stimulus made these cells change their behavior?

We were fortunate, at this time, to enlist the help of a pathology postdoc, already working in our medical school, who had heard about our work and became interested, thinking that this might become his niche in cellular research. She was right and collaborated with us for the next twenty years, after which she was recruited by another university to continue ocular pathology research.

As we kept our patients informed about our laboratory research through quarterly letters, many of them took a keen interest in our progress, especially concerning diabetes. One such patient, Natalie Mosley, was a slightly overweight middle-aged adult-onset diabetic, whose husband had died in a car crash two years before. She was now living with her unmarried thirty-year-old son, who had a secure job with Amtrak as manager of a small suburban railway station on the line from New York to Albany. The job did not pay much, but his mother had no income, supporting herself only on the hundred-thousand-dollar life insurance policy from her husband's job. She was still in her fifties, so that Medicare had not started yet for her. Still, every time she came to the office, she gave me a dollar bill for research.

Natalie especially valued her vision, since she was an artist, an oil painter. On several occasions, she had already temporarily lost her vision, first in one eye, then in both. This was due to hemorrhage into the vitreous cavity. The bleeding was fortunately not severe and cleared up in a few weeks, after which I used the argon laser to obliterate some of the leaking vessels. All this worried her immensely because it threatened her painting career. She really depended partly on the income she derived from the occasional painting that she sold. Besides, painting was what she loved to do.

Other than her eye problems, Natalie was also struggling with her diabetic control. Being overweight made it more difficult, and being the cook in the house, she did not wish to impose a strict diabetic diet on her son. As a result, her blood sugar was high much of the time, which she tried to manage by adjusting her insulin dosage daily. At least twice she passed out and had to be admitted to the hospital in insulin shock, an overdose of insulin. Her blood pressure was also high and fluctuant, which her son had noted when he, as recommended by her diabetologists, took her blood pressure every evening. Several times, when she had developed a serious frontal headache, her pressure was so high that he took her to the emergency room.

"Please, Mom, when you get that headache, call me. You know I don't work far from here."

"Yes, dear boy" was her quiet answer.

A few months later, it was Natalie and her son in the waiting room. He was holding her hand. I had not expected them and double-checked the patient list. She was not on it. After a short wait, I was able to work her into the schedule. Apparently, she had experienced a bad headache followed by some dizziness and then a bilateral sudden loss of vision. First, her vision became red and then black. I assumed that she had hemorrhages in both eyes, which I confirmed during the exam. Her blood pressure was 150/90. I told them to go home and to let Natalie rest, listen to the radio or TV, and sleep with her head up on the pillows.

"And please continue to take your regular meds. Don't fiddle around with your insulin dosage and stick to your diet!"

Her son then told me he could arrange for a daytime caretaker, a neighbor and close friend. That evening, I called Natalie. The neighbor answered the phone and assured me that everything was under control.

A week later, I again saw mother and son in the office. She was supporting herself on his arm as they walked to the exam room, but her pace was not slow. He was carrying a large package under his arm. The exam showed that some of the blood had now settled, at least in one eye, and that her vision had improved to 20/200. She was optimistic and shared her opinion that things were getting much better and that soon, after the blood had cleared, I could simply do a little more laser treatment and fix her up just fine.

Now, her son spoke up.

"But she did want to give you this."

He shoved the package toward me, wrapped in newspaper. I started to unwrap it. "It's her last painting. She did it just last month."

"Please take it. I hope you can hang it in the office. I just want you to have it, in case it really turns out to be my last painting ever. This is why you kept me seeing . . . so I can paint."

As she spoke, a tear rolled down on her cheek. I reached forward and hugged her. It was a lovely moment. The picture was a very colorful still life of an abalone shell on a tablecloth, with iridescent reds, purples, blues, and greens seeming to jump off the canvas. It could have been painted in the seventeenth century by one of the Dutch masters and is, today, still hanging in my old office.

During the following six months, Natalie's vision improved, as I documented several times. Then, on a morning when she did not have an appointment, I spotted her son in the waiting room. He was anxious and had let the desk clerk know that he needed to see me right away. I immediately went over to him and let him follow me to an empty exam room. He was carrying a small Styrofoam cooler with a Lions' Club logo on it, which he put on his lap when he sat down.

"I'm so sorry to bother you, Doctor, but this is so important. Mother died last night. She had a major stroke and never made it to the hospital alive. So I did what she had always wanted. I immediately called the Lions' eye bank to tell them that there was a donor at the Baptist Hospital. They then were able to get her eyes removed in the morgue, put them on dry ice, and give them to me so I could give them to you for your research. This had all been prearranged years before with the Lions' Club. This was what she wanted to do. She really believed in your research and was always sorry that she couldn't give more money. But her eyes were something that she could give. So here they are."

Chapter 2

GROWING UP FAST

In 1960, after internship and a few months of ophthalmic basic science and research at Harvard, I had the opportunity to spend two months in West Africa. John F. Kennedy was president and his brother-in-law, Sargent Shriver, was beginning to talk about the Peace Corps. It was a time of relative quiet in West Africa, but strife had been recent with the change from colonial rule to independence in many nations. As is true after many such revolutions, strife would again return, as competing factions and tribes fought for dominance. As these changes were occurring, America and Russia were also competing for influence in the area. Our pilot project to West Africa was clearly part of the American effort to put its best foot forward.

Two hundred American students, mostly in college, participated. We were divided into ten groups of twenty students each and dispersed to ten different countries, from Senegal to Nigeria. My group went to French-speaking Guinea, a poor country, made even poorer by the French, who, as they departed, destroyed much of the country's infrastructure in angry retaliation for Guinea's choice of total independence from France.

After a couple of days of orientation at the university in Dakar, Senegal, our group took the $1-1/_2$-hour flight to Conakry, the capital of Guinea, where we were met by members of the USIS staff, the

W. A. J. VAN HEUVEN, M.D.

United States Information Service, which ran a small library, where anyone could go to learn about America. We were then loaded into a bus, which transported us more than one hundred miles eastward on partially paved rural roads, to the small inland town of Mamou, where we would be for the next few weeks. Our assigned task was to join a group of Guinean students, roughly the same age, and start building a school for the town.

Mamou, a town of about twenty-five thousand people, was set in the Fouta Djallon rolling hills of rocky terrain and cleared fields, where peanuts were grown. On the edge of town, near a brook, there were also small groups of banana trees. The center of town consisted of a dirt street, less than one mile long, lined with one-story shops. Each shop had a wooden frame and was raised some three feet from the ground. The front part was an open porch, behind which double or triple doors opened into the shop itself. The walls looked like plywood, and the roof was corrugated metal. On almost every balcony was a chair occupied by a male African, who was sewing on a Singer sewing machine. Interestingly, most shopkeepers inside were not African—rather, Lebanese. The street scene was almost entirely pedestrian, with only an occasional small truck. Scantily clad children darted about, men swaggered in their flowing white kaftans and white slippers, and women provided the color, with their beautiful long gowns and head scarfs. They were quite a contrast to our shorts, tennis shoes, and T-shirts.

There were several dirt side streets up-and downhill, lined by trees and brush, among which small clusters of huts stood. Although there were some wooden houses with metal roofs, many living quarters were made of dried mud and straw and were circular, with a steep straw roof starting about five feet from the ground and rising to a peak at least fifteen feet high. There were often no windows. Light came from a round hole at the peak of the roof as well as the front door opening. Many of these homes were small, with a diameter of no more than six meters, but there were also some much larger structures, similarly built, which towered over the others and might have served as communal gathering places. I visited a few of these,

THE EYE: WINDOW TO BODY AND SOUL

where a fire seemed to be constantly maintained in the center, with the smoke rising and exiting through the roof opening. In some side streets, most houses were cement, painted white with rectangular openings for windows—some with shutters—and metal roofs. On both sides of the main street there were also many rocky, at times steep, footpaths leading to other houses, which seemed not to be reachable by any vehicle. It was amazing and wonderful to watch people, often women, negotiate these paths gracefully, carrying large loads on their heads, without any help from their hands. Once I even saw a woman coming down a steep path carrying a bowl of hot tea on her head, without touching the bowl with either hand—a beautiful study of color, balance, and grace.

While we were in Mamou, our quarters were quite comfortable. The girls stayed in a wooden house with several bedrooms and a large living room, where we all ate. Two local women prepared the food in the kitchen, which had electricity. The guys slept in an abandoned cement police station, which consisted of two large rooms with metal army-style beds and a few chairs. We also had electricity and running water but had been warned that it might be contaminated by schistosome parasites, which could enter the body through the skin. We were thus very careful not to let the water touch the skin very long. We never really bathed and rigged up a shower outside. A water filter provided safe drinking water.

One day, after we had returned from the countryside, where we had been gathering rocks for the school's foundation and transporting them by small truck, a young boy, probably around twelve years old, came to our quarters and asked who the doctor was. He was accompanied by two younger girls. He spoke French and had heard that one of the visiting Americans was a doctor. He asked me if I would follow him to his home. His father had sent him, he told me, because one of his younger sisters had an eye problem.

"Quelle sorte de problème?" I asked.

"Elle est aveugle!" (She is blind!) he exclaimed, throwing his hands up.

"I'm not sure I'll be able to do too much, but I'll follow you. Let's see what it is."

We went up a small path near our quarters and came to an adobe hut where several other children were playing, and a young man was standing by the door opening, as if waiting for something. The boy kept talking to me, "Ce n'est pas loin, nous sommes presque la." (It's not far, we're almost there.) Meanwhile, the girls were talking to one another in Fulah, or at least it sounded to me like the language most of the Mamou people spoke.

"This is my father," he stated as we approached the waiting man. "And he speaks French. He'll tell you all about Angélique."

The man stepped forward. He formally stretched out his hand and, with a small bow, shook mine.

"*Merci, merci, merci* for coming. Sorry to bother you, but when I heard that you were a doctor, I just had to get you to look at my seven-year-old daughter. Can anything be done?"

Then, turning to his son, he said, "Maruf, go get her. She's inside."

The boy came back walking slowly and was holding a little girl by the hand. She looked like she was no more than five years old and quite thin. Her eyes were closed.

"Does she ever open her eyes?" I asked.

"No, not really. Inside the house maybe, but never outside. The light seems to hurt her, so she says."

"Let me take a look. Does she speak French?"

"Oh yes, I made sure of that. All the boys and a couple of the girls speak French. Their mothers don't, but these days I think that all children have to learn French, especially the boys, just to get along."

"How many children do you have?"

"Right now, eleven, and I think that's it!" Then he quickly added, "But I have four wives." He smiled. "You Westerners must think that's very complicated, but we're used to that."

I sat down on a tree stump and took Angélique's hand so that she stood facing me, between my knees, her face within easy reach. I put my hands on her temples and stroked them softly.

"Angélique, can you open your eyes, *ma chérie*?" She complied, her eyelids trembling. I got a quick glance at her pupils. They were constricted and small in the bright light but totally white, obviously due to dense cataracts.

"Would you be more comfortable inside, where it is a little darker?" She nodded yes. Inside the hut, I sat down on a small bench and again faced her, standing between my knees.

"I know that you know where I am, but can you see where my head is? Try touching my ear or my nose or chin." She hesitated but then reached forward and put her fingers awkwardly on my cheek.

"Very good." I wondered if she really saw something, but I persisted.

"Now I am going to hold my hands in front of both of your eyes, and tell me if it gets darker. Then I will take my hands away, and you can then tell me if it gets a little lighter. I'm going to start now. If at any time it gets a tiny bit lighter, let me know. Whenever you see any change, just say 'darker' or 'lighter.' Do you understand?"

She nodded.

"Just keep your eyes open."

At first, she said nothing. Then she spoke up: "*Oui, oui,* a little lighter, and now it's black again."

The game continued for several minutes until I was convinced that she did have the ability to differentiate light from dark.

"Angélique, you are wonderful. I am going to come back in a few days and bring some of my special lights so I can find out if I can help you or not." I kissed her on the cheek, and she, surprised, again touched my face with her fingers. I then explained to her father what I was doing. I would be back as soon as I could get my hands on some pupil-dilating drugs.

A few days later, I had a small bottle of homatropine, which the midwife at the local dispensary was able to get from a pharmacy in Conakry. It came by mail bus and took two days to get to Mamou. At the end of that day, I again went to see Angélique. She was outside her home, sitting on the ground and playing with a small ball. I helped her up and, holding one hand, went inside, while her father and several of the other children were watching. Besides the homatropine, I also had brought my small doctor's black bag, which had not left my side since my fourth year in medical school. Other than a stethoscope, it also contained a penlight and some anesthetic eye drops. First, I anesthetized her cornea and conjunctiva so that I could place the penlight directly on the white of her eyes.

"Tell me if you see any light at any time."

It was a suspenseful moment. I turned on the small bright light, and her reaction was instantaneous.

"*Oui, oui, oui*, I can see a light, very bright!"

"Fantastic."

I then tested all quadrants of both eyes, and the response was the same.

"Well, I think that the back part of both eyes seems to be working. Now I am going to use some special eye drops from Conakry, which will dilate her pupils and maybe let some light in. The drops will take about half an hour to work, so I am going home right now, and I'll be back in twenty minutes. Meanwhile, just keep her inside."

What I was trying to figure out was whether the girl's congenital cataracts consisted of white opacities in the entire lens of each eye or just in the central part, a so-called nuclear cataract. In retrospect, my thinking was somewhat premature, since I had not even had a single day of ophthalmology training in my life and had never seen a congenital cataract. Most of my rudimentary knowledge had come from my ophthalmologist father, who had specifically talked about congenital cataracts. That conversation occurred because when we still lived in the Netherlands, one of the daughters of Queen Juliana was born with cataracts. It was national news and certainly was part of the conversation among Dutch ophthalmologists. My father had told me about the different types of cataract, some with complete opacification of the lens and some with only partial whitening. For a while, he had even brought some cataractous lenses, which he had removed from patients, home with him so that we could dissect them on our plates at the end of lunch. It was a fascinating activity, which our kitchen maid did not seem to appreciate, especially when the dissected specimen came back to the kitchen.

When I returned twenty minutes later, Angélique's pupils were well dilated. Her eyes were open, and she was looking all around, as if she had discovered a new world. I am sure that she still could not see clearly, but she was walking around touching things, not needing help to steer her.

"So that's you. I can see you," I heard her say several times, as she visually met some of her siblings for the first time. The little kids did not know what to make of it. They had never experienced her like this before. I believe they still thought that she needed to hold their hands to lead her.

"No, I'm okay, I can do it. I can do it."

It was a breakthrough moment, also for me, because now I knew what should be done next. I checked her again with my penlight, and when I placed it on the white of her eye, I could see the central nuclear cataracts surrounded by a halo of light coming back through the pupil, like the halo of light surrounding a total eclipse of the sun. I explained it to her father and told him that we were going to keep her pupils dilated until I could make some arrangements with an eye surgeon. I suggested that the family start treating her like a normal child, although her vision, even dilated, was still very poor. I believe that he understood.

During the next three weeks, I visited the family daily, making certain that the drops were given regularly. The father told me that Angélique was a changed child, having gone from meek and reticent to outgoing and excited. She wanted to touch everything and everyone. While looking at her family and friends, she would often feel their faces with both hands, saying, "Don't say anything. I'll tell you who you are."

She had also started to eat more, even more than her ten-year-old brother, as if she was trying to catch up. I asked her father, "Do you think that the other kids had been stealing food off her plate?"

"I don't know." He shrugged.

Meanwhile, I had convinced our group leader that removing the cataracts on this girl might have a very positive effect on this town, perhaps even more important than starting to build a school. Were we not there in Guinea to demonstrate that Americans had a great interest in promoting its image, after the French had left it so destitute? He agreed, and we formed a plan to find a well-trained ophthalmic surgeon to operate. With the help of the USIS library staff in Conakry, with whom we spoke multiple times, using the police station telephone, an arrangement was made to transfer Angélique to the French military hospital in Dakar, Senegal. Every two months, an ophthalmologist from Paris would come to Dakar for a few days to examine and then operate on patients with a variety of eye conditions. If we let him know in advance about the congenital cataract, he would be prepared.

It was my job to accompany Angélique to Dakar, a short flight from Conakry. The father agreed to the plan and signed a few documents in approval. Two weeks later, a USIS van picked us up in Mamou. Two hours later, we were at Conakry airport for the short flight to Dakar. There, another USIS employee took us to the hospital, which was ready to receive us. Angélique was given a bed in a semiprivate room with an armchair for me. I spent the rest of the day and evening with her so that she would not feel alone in this strange environment and then went to sleep in a doctor's on-call room. The next morning, I joined Angélique again until she was taken to the operating suite. Apparently, the doctor had decided to do both eyes at the same time, given the circumstances. This was rarely done in the Western world because of the fear that an infection due to an inadvertent break in sterile technique, if it occurred, might infect both eyes.

The operations went well and gave Angélique immediate and fantastic improvement in her vision, especially when she was given a pair of temporary thick +14.00 diopter glasses. She could barely believe what she could see. It was gratifying to watch her elation.

She spent the next three days in the hospital getting eye drops frequently and exploring the hallways. The nurses loved her attitude and cheerful, outgoing personality and often invited her to sit with them in the nurse's station. It was good for Angélique to have all these "mothers" around and also easier for them to keep an eye on her and give her the drops. It also permitted me to take a few hours every day to roam around Dakar, a touristy city with restaurants and nice shops, which seemed more Western than African. I even spent one afternoon at a French hotel on the beach, which was obviously a resort frequented by white-skinned Frenchmen.

On the fourth postop day, when the surgeon was planning to return to Paris, I met with him in the early morning and was given instructions to take our patient back to Conakry, where I would make certain that she would continue her eye drops for at least six weeks. He asked if there was an ophthalmologist anywhere in Guinea, where she might get her glasses prescription redone. I promised to find out.

"She can really see. It's fantastic. Now we must teach her to read and write, just like her brothers. She already speaks French, not like the other girls and their mothers. With those glasses, she already looks like she's educated. She looks like a teacher, like a professor. Maybe she can become a doctor. Why not an eye doctor!"

In his excitement, her father had already planned her whole life. Angélique just smiled.

During the next few weeks, I saw Angélique daily to look at her with my penlight. Her father was giving the eye drops, and the eyes began to look less red and felt more comfortable, so she said. Her brother Maruf had taken it upon himself to start teaching her to read. She was a fast and enthusiastic learner, which kindled even more excitement for both student and teacher. Pretty soon, the other girls, who barely spoke French, also wanted to learn more. The whole family almost became a school in itself, with the father in charge.

"I guess we are all going to be educated," he commented, obviously proud of this decision.

Six weeks following surgery, the father took Angélique to Conakry by bus to see an Egyptian ophthalmologist, whom I had heard about. They came back with a new pair of glasses, a smaller horn-rimmed frame with a refined prescription, which improved the vision even more. Two weeks later, our group left Guinea to return home, via Dakar and Paris. The foundation of the school had been finished, and walls were being erected. It was fall.

The next spring, I wrote a letter to the father, asking about Angélique. In the late fall, probably after things in Mamou had quieted down following the peanut harvest, I got a response. It was a short letter thanking me again for arranging the surgery and finding such a fantastic French doctor to do it. He also included a picture of Angélique and himself in front of their hut. She now looked her age. Both were smiling.

During the next three years, we communicated yearly. The school building was completed, and Angélique became a regular student. She excelled in French and had caught up to her classmates, who were mostly boys. She had started teaching French and reading to her own sisters. She was happy. The last letter, when she was ten, she had written herself.

"This is the first letter I have ever written. I am so glad to be able to write it to you. This would never have happened without you. *Merci, merci, mon docteur.* I hope you are well."

Several years passed before the next letter. It was now ten years since Mamou, during which time I had moved several times while finishing my medical education. The letter took three months to get to me. It was very brief but included a picture of three adults standing next to one another in front of a hut: a young man; a beautifully and colorfully dressed young woman with a headscarf and glasses, holding a baby in her arms; and the father. The young man had his arm around her shoulder, and the father had a small American flag in his left hand. They were all smiling. The note stated, "I thought that you might want to meet my husband and see our baby. We are very happy. *Tout va bien.*"

Chapter 3

I'll Forever Love You

Czetnerovski, Rebecca, diabetes was the next entry on the patient list. Polish names were not uncommon in Upstate New York. Most Poles had come during the start-up of the garment mills during the mid-eighteen hundreds and had settled there to take the many jobs, both for men and women, which were available. As a result, many families had two incomes, which produced a solid basis for a middle-class existence.

Rebecca was already sitting on the exam chair when I entered the room. She was a small girl with unkempt long hair hiding most of her face. She was looking down and did not move when I entered. She seemed diminutive in the large chair, with her arms tight against her body, with hands folded on her lap. It seemed like she really did not want to be in a doctor's office.

On another chair sat a young man with a very different demeanor. He was a sportily dressed, good-looking blond blue-eyed seventeen-year-old who looked up at me right away. He sat on the edge of his chair, leaning toward me, ready to start speaking.

"I am Joe Petrovski. I'm Rebecca's friend. Doctor, let me tell you why we are here. Yesterday, Rebecca suddenly went blind. It happened after she had walked to the end of the driveway to pick up the mail. We were sitting at the kitchen table, and she started blinking her eyes. She said that she couldn't see."

"Both eyes at the same time?" I asked.

She answered slowly, still looking down. "First . . . it seemed that it was in both eyes, but now I think it was mostly on the left side, because I already had some trouble seeing out of the right eye before. That had already been that way for several months, but I thought it would clear up. I really never mentioned it to anyone, not even to him," She turned her head toward Joe. "Sorry, dear, I just didn't want to worry you."

Now I could see her face for the first time. She was not a pretty girl, with pale gray skin, heavy eyebrows, and some chin hairs. She was frowning, with deep furrows on her forehead. She wore no makeup. My eye exam was short, and dilating drops were used right away. Her vision was poor, unable to see any letters on the chart. She was, however, able to see my hand movements in both eyes. The right eye was full of dark blood, but the blood in the left eye was still red, indicating a fresh bleed. She told me about her health, how she had had diabetes since age six and had taken insulin ever since. The diabetes had been difficult to control early on, but now that she was older, she had figured it out, as long as she continued to take insulin four times a day.

"Joe here has really helped me with getting the right dose. He knows me so well that he can tell whether I have had too much or too little. I now have very few insulin reactions. Back when I was ten or twelve, I had them all the time. Even then Joe was helping me."

"You've known each other that long?" I asked.

Joe answered, "We have been like brother and sister since she was four and I was six. First, we were neighbors, and then my father and her mother died the same year, one of acute leukemia and the other of a brain tumor. Totally unrelated. It was awful. And so a year later, our surviving parents married each other. That was fantastic. We've all been living together ever since."

He looked up at me and smiled. Then he looked at her. "And so I've been taking care of my little sister ever since."

She was now also smiling. "It's true. He has been my savior."

"You've been so lucky to have such a caring brother. I also know of some other brothers who would never lift a finger to help their siblings. Instead they just competed with them."

We then discussed what should be done next to make Rebecca see again. First, she should see her diabetes doctor to make sure she was stable.

"Is your blood pressure ok?"

"I think so. I'm taking medicine for it."

"Then your doctor should also make sure that it is also under good control. If you tell me his name, I shall call him and tell him what we are planning."

"It's Dr. Peter Adams. Do you know him?"

"Yes, very well. He's very good. After he checks you, I'll schedule you for some surgery. I can remove blood from both eyes and see what the retina looks like. I am guessing that your left retina will look pretty good, since your bleed was very recent. Then we'll see about the other eye."

After Rebecca and Joe left, I called Peter Adams right away. We talked for several minutes, with both of us recognizing the difference we could make in this girl's life.

Rebecca's situation reminded me of Betsy, a patient whom I had seen a year before, another young girl with a similar story of childhood-onset diabetes and poor blood sugar control. She had become blind in both eyes at age twenty, just after finishing high school. She was obese, weighing over 250 pounds, and paid little attention to her diet. She had had a confrontational relationship with her single mother, who had tried to control her daughter to little avail. Emergency room (ER) visits were frequent, the usual cause being an insulin overdose. Betsy was an obstinate person, but when her blood sugar dropped, she became quite obstreperous, even refusing to take some orange juice, which might have avoided the hospital visit. She had an independent streak and thus, as soon as school was finished, had moved in with her boyfriend, who seemed to have no idea how to handle her.

When she lost her vision from bilateral diabetic intraocular hemorrhages, she came to the ER. Her blood sugar was 180 (high), and her blood pressure was 170/110, high enough for her to be admitted to the hospital. Ophthalmology was consulted.

Our exam, done in the ER without the benefit of some of our usual instrumentation, showed very poor vision, probably caused by severe intraocular blood. I recommended vitrectomy surgery (removal of the vitreous gel together with the blood) as soon as her medical condition was stabilized. A week later, before she was discharged, I operated on both eyes three days apart. Her vision improved immediately, and we could now see her severe diabetic as well as hypertensive retinopathy. She must have had high blood pressure for a long time, which was surprising to me, since she had supposedly been under a doctor's care for most of her life. When she was discharged, her insulin dose had been changed, and blood pressure medication was prescribed.

Two weeks later, she was back in the ER with another insulin reaction. Her blood pressure was again dangerously high, and her vision in one eye had again worsened. The patient insisted that she had taken her pills.

"I may have forgotten once," she had said nonchalantly.

We were again consulted. Her vision in the right eye had decreased slightly, but now she had a branch retinal vein occlusion, a complication of high blood pressure.

"You have had a small stroke in your eye. It's due to blood pressure. You've got to take your pills. Don't forget. The blood vessel in your retina, which became obstructed, was fortunately only a small branch. But next time, it could be a bigger vessel. You could lose much of your vision in that eye, and that would be permanent. There's no treatment for that stuff. We can only try to prevent it by controlling your blood pressure. Do you understand?"

She nodded, as did her boyfriend, who had brought her in.

"Perhaps you can help make sure that she takes her pills," I said, turning to him.

"I'll try, but I'm not with her all the time. I have a full-time job."

"Do what you can."

THE EYE: WINDOW TO BODY AND SOUL

A few minutes later, the internal medicine resident came and again explained her diet and insulin dosage and how to prevent the insulin reactions leading to ER visits. The boyfriend listened intently.

"I know all that stuff" was Betsy's comment. After that, she was allowed to go home.

Two months later, there was another insulin reaction and ER visit. Her high blood pressure again forced a hospital admission. This time she was found to be pregnant, having gained another ten pounds. The blood pressure took several days to control, during which we were again consulted. Her vision had now decreased in both eyes, not from vitreous hemorrhage but from retinal edema, swelling of the retina due to the high blood pressure. This was a classic case of preeclampsia, which might even result in bilateral retinal detachments.

We spoke with the obstetrician and the internist, both of whom recommended terminating the pregnancy. Betsy refused and signed herself out of the hospital against doctor's advice. Her boyfriend picked her up with the comment, "What can *I* do?"

We did not see her for several months. Then I got a call from the internist to tell me that Betsy had suffered a major stroke, was admitted, and died two days later in the intensive care unit. Her baby was too premature to save.

I could not get away from the thought that Betsy's story was very similar to Rebecca's. Both were young girls with juvenile diabetes and hypertension, difficult to control medically. Both were at risk for pregnancy. However, Rebecca seemed to have a better support system, which might make it easier for me to be successful. Certainly, I promised myself to do everything possible not to fail again and to prevent Rebecca from ending up with the same fate as Betsy.

It took a few weeks to get Rebecca ready for surgery. Her diabetic control was fine-tuned, and her blood pressure medicine was adjusted. There were no other medical problems uncovered. A pregnancy test was negative. Joe was her constant companion at every office visit.

I operated on the left eye first, performing a so-called vitrectomy, and was able to remove most of the red blood. Her vision instantly improved to 20/30. The retina, from which the bleeding had occurred, showed some abnormal blood vessels which, on angiography, proved to be the bleeding source. These I treated with laser to prevent future bleeding. Then I did a vitrectomy on the right eye. Again the blood, which was clotted and dark, was removed successfully. Laser was done to leaky vessels, but there was considerable scarring on the retina surface, making the probability of good vision less. Her vision improved to 20/200, the big *E* on the chart. Chances of further improvement seemed slim. Notwithstanding that limited success, Rebecca and Joe were elated and thanked me profusely. She was like a changed person and was no longer reticent and depressed.

During the subsequent two years, I saw them both every three months. On two occasions, I had to perform more laser to control small hemorrhages. Her diabetes and hypertension were now better controlled than ever, thanks to Peter Adams, who was seeing them every three months as well.

At the last visit, Rebecca and Joe seemed especially ebullient. She also looked different. Her hair was pulled back into a ponytail, her facial hairs were gone, her skin was tanned and lustrous, and she wore some lipstick and small pearl earrings. It was the first time that I saw her as being quite pretty. They could hardly wait to tell me that they had decided to get married. They joked about some of their friends who did not know their family history, and they had asked, How could you marry your own sister? That was supposed to be illegal! My reaction was positive. I congratulated them on their decision and hugged them both.

"Together I know that you will keep this diabetes under control. You are very lucky, Rebecca, to have Joe and also to not have some of the other problems of diabetes, such as kidney or circulation problems. If you don't do anything to upset the apple cart, you'll live forever. By the way, have you discussed having children?"

Rebecca answered, "I'm glad you asked. Joe and I talked to Dr. Adams about that. He thought that would not be a good idea. He was pretty firm about it. He put me on a pill to prevent pregnancy. He said that my blood pressure might just go through the roof if I got pregnant. He scared me enough, so I am taking the pill right now. Still, I would love to have a baby. What do *you* think?"

"I must say, I agree completely with Dr. Adams. Let me tell you a story."

I then told them the sad story of Betsy and how committed I was not to let that ever happen again to anybody.

"I see that as a failure on my part. I really never got to know Betsy well enough to have an influence. I should have tried harder so that she would listen to me. I know that's not going to happen with you, Rebecca. We've come a long way already, and I'm not going to let you out of my sight."

After that comment, Rebecca got up, leaned forward, and kissed me on the cheek.

Four months later, I got the invitation to their wedding. It was held at a small inn on a lake north of town. Peter Adams and I were the only invitees without a Polish last name. Rebecca looked beautiful and graceful. Joe looked strong. They articulated their vows audibly and confidently.

During the next couple of years, the regular visits with Peter Adams and me continued every three months. We again started to talk about babies. I told her that one of my own two children was adopted, which surprised them and seemed to make them recognize that adoption was a real option for them.

"Just make sure that you know something about the parents, and also get the child medically checked. You don't need a sick child. You've got enough to do taking care of yourself."

During the following year, I put Rebecca and Joe in touch with the local Catholic Charities organization, through which my wife and I had adopted our second son many years before. I was able to meet with the same lady, Mrs. Beasly, who had helped us. She immediately understood the importance, in this case, of the child being healthy. She found a five-month-old blond boy, son of a sixteen-year-old single mother, who tried but was unable to care for him. He had already been at five foster homes when he was finally given to Catholic Charities. I accompanied Rebecca and Joe to their first meeting with the child, which was highly successful. The boy never cried and smiled and giggled as Rebecca held him.

"It's a marriage made in heaven," I mused. "The child even looks Polish."

After the meeting, I asked Mrs. Beasly if I could arrange a thorough physical exam for the boy before any final decision was made. She agreed. During the next ten days, I had him examined by a pediatrician, by a cardiologist, and by me. All examinations were normal, including a dilated eye exam. After that, the paperwork was quickly completed, and the adoption took place. The child's name, which had been David, now became David Joseph Petrovski, using his adoptive father's first name.

During the next several years, I stayed in close contact with the family. The three-month visits were amplified by periodic phone calls. My excuse for calling was that I was not going to let her out of my sight. And so I watched David grow up and saw him go to kindergarten and first grade, and I did his second eye exam, which was again normal. It was almost like examining one of my own children.

"I can't thank you enough. You have made all this possible. We should call you Grandpa. We are so happy!"

With that, Rebecca stood up on her tiptoes, kissed me on the cheek, and whispered, "I'll forever love you."

Chapter 4

Dependence

Right away, I took a dislike to Helen Cartwright. She was just another patient who was diabetic, obese, and on disability, all because she had not taken care of herself. She was forty-six years old and was living with her father, who had just started getting social security and Medicare, so there was at least some income to support them. Her mother had died several years before of diabetic complications, so she should have learned something from that experience, I thought. She waddled slowly into the exam room and sat down where I indicated.

"Hello, Doctor, I'm here because of my diabetes, I guess. My diabetic doctor told me to see you." Her voice was high-pitched but soft, like a meek child, not yet past puberty.

"My daddy also wanted me to see an eye doctor. He heard about how diabetes can make you blind, but I can see just fine. He's always worried about me. I don't know why. I take good care of him, I clean, I cook, I shop. He loves it all. I'm Daddy's girl, so he still worries about me."

"Maybe because of your diabetes, maybe because of your being overweight. Maybe because you are disabled. How are you disabled anyway, if you can do all these things for your, uh, daddy?"

"Well, it is because I keep passing out. Recently, my doctor put me on insulin, and sometimes I get too much of it depending on how

I eat. I have a lot of trouble figuring what or when to eat. I seem to be hungry all the time. Then, some days, when I eat almost no sugar, I get what my doctors tells me is an insulin reaction. I get very upset, sweaty, and then very weak. For the last month alone, I have had three of them. Twice, my daddy had to call an ambulance. Once they kept me overnight in the hospital. Daddy says he can often predict when it's about to happen, because I get fidgety and nasty and I refuse to drink the orange juice he gives me."

"Let's look at your eyes and see what you've got." I pushed the slit lamp toward her and asked her to put her chin on the chin rest. She obliged, and I started the exam. The tech had already taken her vision, which was 20/20 without glasses. I assumed that the glasses, which hung on a cord around her neck, were for reading. As the exam progressed, I kept the discussion going. She told me about her mother dying at a young age and also about her most recent job, helping her father's friend in a neighborhood bakery.

"Do you get paid for what you do at the bakery?"

"No, not really . . . Actually just a little bit, but I get some free food."

"A lot of sweets, I bet." "I guess."

"Maybe that's not the best place for you to work." She nodded.

As I finished the exam, which was essentially normal, I began to wonder how to approach this person, who was doing wrong things to take care of herself. If her father ever became disabled or would die, what kind of future would she have? How could she cope on her own? Could she ever be independent?

"You're very lucky so far. You have no diabetic damage in your eyes, but that could change any time. You really must lose weight to begin with. How much do you weigh right now?"

"A hundred and eighty-four pounds this morning, but my blood sugar was good, barely over a hundred."

"Does your diabetes doctor have a plan for you?"

"He's trying to start me on a diet, but he hasn't given it to me yet."

"Who is your doctor anyway?"

"It's Dr. Jorge Gonzalez, downstairs, right in this building."

THE EYE: WINDOW TO BODY AND SOUL

"I'm going to talk to him about you, if that's all right."

"Of course." She smiled.

That afternoon, after all patients had left, I called Dr. Gonzalez. I vented my frustration about all these patients we had who were in a similar predicament: diabetes and obesity and then, in some cases, blindness.

"And then, if they just lost weight and got control of their metabolism, they might not even have diabetes at all."

He agreed, and we both decided that this girl would be a perfect target for our joint efforts to get her well. He would get her an appointment with a nutritionist, and we would insist that the patient bring her father to her next appointments.

The following day, I telephoned the patient's home, and the father answered. I told him that Dr. Gonzalez and I were worried about his daughter and that he could help us get her on the right path. He would have to help with the new diet that he, too, should learn about by accompanying her to the nutritionist. I also suggested that no one in his house should eat anything after 7:00 PM. Instead, after dinner, he and she should take a one-hour walk. He should also not let her do the shopping by herself.

"Don't give her the money, but go with her. You pay the bill. Also, it's probably not good for her to be working in your friend's bakery. Do you think you can stop that?"

"I'll try."

"Do so, and please come with your daughter to her next appointment with me."

Two months later, they came to my office together.

"Here, I want you to meet my daddy. He insisted that he come along." Her voice was again like that of a child, high-pitched and without overtones.

"Pleasure to meet you, sir. I'm glad you came. Are there things going on since we spoke on the telephone?"

"You talked to each other before?" she piped up. "I didn't know that."

I nodded. "And we had a wonderful conversation. It was all about eating the right food so that you'll lose some weight and maybe prevent some of the diabetic eye problems. Tell me what you two have accomplished so far," I said, turning to the father.

"Actually, quite a bit! We've gotten all the new diet information and have seen the nutritionist already three times. We are following it pretty darn well. Me too. It's even made me lost a couple of pounds. And my little honey bee here, that's what I call her, is also losing weight. Three pounds so far. She weighs herself every morning and eats nothing after supper, and then we take our walk, just like you suggested, Doctor. Then, when we come home from that, we watch the same stupid TV show, some British comedy, just to distract us enough so we don't graze the refrigerator. It all seems to work. And it's been fun. We are spending a lot of time together."

She was smiling as he spoke and then told me that she had not had any insulin reactions for two months and had not adjusted her insulin at all recently as she used to do almost daily when her diet was erratic.

The eye exam that day was essentially normal, with no evidence of diabetic retina involvement. Her vision was 20/20. As they were leaving, she said, "Oh, Doctor. I haven't told you the most exciting thing. I'm not going to the bakery any more. They didn't really need me anyway, but I found a part-time job, working right here in this building in the nutrition and diet office. I'm sort of a receptionist, greeting patients, getting them to the right nurses, handing out diet instructions, and all that. Dr. Gonzalez helped arrange it. And so now, I'm not on disability anymore. Isn't that great? Isn't that what you wanted?"

"Absolutely, and congratulations! Let me tell you that you've surprised me a little bit. I didn't have much confidence that you would really listen to me and start changing your life. So congratulations again!"

"Thank you, Doctor, but it wasn't just you. Dr. Gonzalez helped, and then the nutritionist, and then . . . there is my daddy. I always need my daddy."

THE EYE: WINDOW TO BODY AND SOUL

They left with an appointment for three months. I told them that would be fine, since her eyes were as of yet not affected by the diabetes, but I warned them that I might call before that time to make sure that progress was continuing.

Two months later, I called her. She was doing well, enjoying the time with her father and loving her job, which had become full-time. Still, her big problem was hunger. She was always hungry and had, on many days, gone off her diet to sneak in a few bites of sweets. All she had to do was to go across the street to the local bank, where there was a huge bowl of candy on the counter as you entered.

One month later, the eye exam was again normal. She and her father had come together, and all of us were thankful that the eyes had been spared so far. She had lost fifteen pounds but was still on insulin. She continued to be hungry much of the time and still had difficulty keeping on her diet. At most meals, she ate twice as much as her father. Their evening walks had continued, although they were a little slower now because her father had developed atrial fibrillation, which made him dizzy once in a while. She described how they now held hands as they walked to give him stability.

That afternoon, I called Jorge Gonzalez. After congratulating each other about our success with our mutual patient, he told me two new pieces of information. The first was that he had started to discuss a surgical option with her, a banding of the stomach, which would effectively decrease her stomach size and make her less tolerant of large meals. In fact, patients who had that procedure were often less hungry, especially after only a few bites. He thought that she might be the perfect candidate for the operation, which was not very invasive. He also acknowledged that it didn't always work but might be worth a try. Then he told me that he would be leaving our hospital to take a new job in Houston, which would start the following year.

"So let's get this girl fixed up before then."

I agreed.

During the next few months, Jorge kept me informed about the stomach surgery. It had gone well without complications, and the result was a significant loss of appetite. She had continued to lose weight and no longer needed insulin. Instead, she was taking a diabetic control pill.

"If she keeps this up, she may even stop having diabetes altogether" was his final comment.

"Then she won't need either of us anymore" was my hopeful response.

A few weeks later, just before her next appointment, she telephoned. Because she was still working in the nutrition office, I had seen her several times, greeting her as we passed in the hallway. She had seemed like a changed person, walking energetically, no longer obese, and appearing much younger. I expected her phone call to be about postponing her eye exam, because she was doing so well. Instead, she told me that her father had had a small stroke, which left him very weak on his right side. This made walking difficult, so their evening walks were now curtailed. She hoped that she would not start nibbling again in the evenings. I suggested that she find a friend, maybe a neighbor, to walk with.

"I'll try."

"By the way, make sure you keep your appointment with me so that we can talk some more."

"Yes, I'll be there for sure."

When she returned, her attitude was positive. She and her father had a slightly new routine, and she had found a neighbor, a woman across the street, to walk with at night. Her eye exam showed good vision and no evidence of diabetic retinopathy. She told me that Dr. Gonzalez was slowing down in preparation for his Houston move, but he had decided to taper her off her diabetic medication, since she really didn't have diabetes anymore. He had suggested that she see another doctor perhaps every six months for a while to make certain that her blood sugar stayed under control.

"I'll miss Dr. Gonzalez. He took such good care of me, like another daddy. He was the one who really convinced me to have the stomach surgery."

A few months later, she called me again to tell me about her father's second stroke. It was very severe and put him in the ICU for several days. Then he died in his sleep.

"I'm very sorry to hear that. Tell me how you are coping. What can I do?"

"Oh, nothing now. I'm okay. I knew that this would happen sometime, I guess I was sort of ready for it. But I just needed to talk to you and tell you what happened. I'll be getting used to being by myself. Fortunately, the woman across the street, the one I walk with, has become a very good friend. That'll help."

"Well, you sound okay. Stay on your diet, and you should be fine and without diabetes! You really don't need to see me that often anymore, and I see you in the hall once in a while anyway! Why don't you make an appointment for six months so I can look at your eyes again? Not that I expect to find anything wrong."

"But, Dr. van Heuven, can't I just come see you in about two months? With my father's death and Dr. Gonzalez gone, you're my daddy now."

Chapter 5

Pallbearer

I knew her from church, having spoken to her several times during the coffee hour following the ten o'clock Sunday service. But then, so did everyone else in the Episcopal congregation. She was the beautifully coiffed "grand dame," dressed conservatively but always in the latest fashion, her short white hair pulled back to emphasize a high forehead and an unusual sparsity of wrinkles for a seventy-seven-year-old lady. She wore no glasses, and her bright-blue eyes, like small blue gemstones, accentuated her fine features: a small nose, thin lips, and a child's chin.

She always entered the church through a side door near the altar at the last minute before the service started, when most everyone else was already seated. She was usually accompanied by her daughter, whose hand she let go as they came through the door. After that, she was on her own, looking quickly to the window behind the altar, which had an inscription on it, indicating that she and her now-deceased husband had donated that window to the church many years before. Then, facing the audience, she nodded, doing almost a small curtsy before she strode erectly and confidently to her seat in the first row, just in front of the pulpit. From there, she could easily read the small plaque indicating that it, too, had been donated by her family.

THE EYE: WINDOW TO BODY AND SOUL

During the service, it was hard to tell how much she participated. I presumed that she knew most of it by heart, because from my angle of observation, I could see her jaw move during the prayers and the creeds. Then, whenever we were singing a hymn, she often put on a pair of glasses.

At the postservice coffee, she and her daughter came up to me to ask about ophthalmology.

"I hear you know something about macular degeneration. I have a friend who suggested that I talk to you. My optometrist told me a few months ago that I had it, but I can see just fine. I know that he's not a real doctor."

"It's nice to see you. Do you have an eye doctor other than the optometrist?"

"Not anymore. I used to go to Dr. Shumacher, but he's been dead for years. Doctors should always outlive their patients."

"Well, I do specialize in retinal problems, and I see a lot of patients with macular degeneration. So maybe you would like to see me sometime? I'm at the medical school."

"I don't really know where that is, but my driver will find it, if you give him the proper instructions. I know there's been a lot of development out there during the last forty years, but I just never had to go out there. I stay right here in my neighborhood. We've got everything here—shops, restaurants, the country club, you name it."

"It'll be nice to have you visit the medical school. Let's make it at a special time so that I can give you a short tour of the place. You'll be pleasantly surprised."

"That sounds fine, thank you."

"I'll give you a call to arrange it."

A couple of weeks later, I telephoned her and left a message with her housekeeper. By then, I had found out more about her, that she indeed did, quite often, get out of the neighborhood to fly to Houston for the opera and to New York and even to London for the theater.

When she appeared at the office around 11:00 AM, she was accompanied by her daughter, who had apparently no trouble finding the medical school. She was the last patient of the morning so that

I would have a chance to give her a brief tour afterward. I had also called the president of the medical school to arrange a meeting around 12:30 PM, which I thought might be of mutual benefit to both of them. As she came into the waiting room, she was holding onto her daughter's arm and looking down at the floor, as if she was expecting uneven terrain. I had seen them coming, and when they saw me, the mother straightened her posture and confidently stepped forward toward me, hand outstretched. I welcomed them and introduced them to my clinic manager, an outgoing, well-dressed middle-aged woman who understood that this was a moment to be deferential.

"Welcome to our office. It's so nice to see you. Dr. van Heuven told me you were coming," she said.

"A pleasure to meet you. Your name?"

"Liz Campbell. Just call me Liz." She then took the two women to an exam room.

The eye exam went very efficiently and right away demonstrated significantly decreased vision in one eye. The other eye was 20/20, although she had to guess at some of the letters.

"Were you aware that your vision in your left eye is not as good as the other one?"

"Not really. I can see just fine. I just sometimes have some trouble reading, that's all. I seem to lose my place on the page."

During the retina part of the exam, it became obvious that she had signs of macular degeneration in both eyes, evidenced by pigment disturbances centrally in each retina, particularly in the left eye, where there was an absence of the normal pigment in the very center of the retina, the macula. This was typical of macular atrophy, so-called dry macular degeneration. In the right eye, however, the depigmentation was not central and only barely visible. Retinal pictures were taken, and an angiogram was done, which confirmed the diagnosis. As we all sat down and looked at the photos, I explained what she had, and although she had been unlucky in one eye, it might be many years, if ever, that she would lose more vision in the good eye. It would be important, however, to take a special multivitamin pill, combined with zinc and lutein, every day for the rest of her life. I also showed her a tiny depigmented spot near the center in her right eye, which was probably responsible for her losing her place on the page while reading. I told her how one of my mentors once taught me that patients with early dry macular generation often had those tiny central defects, which he said caused fractured vision.

"But how do you know that I won't lose my vision in the good eye soon?"

"Because this condition, although progressive, is very slow to change. I bet that you have had poor vision in your left eye already for many years. That's what it looks like. And now that you'll be taking these vitamins, it will be even slower. And then, on top of that, I'll be seeing you every three months to take pictures and do an angiogram, which will show us if your type of degeneration is changing—that is, becoming what we call wet. That is a condition that we can treat with a laser."

"I sure hope that you're right, Doctor, and please promise me that you'll outlive me!"

"I promise" was my curt reply. She laughed. A few days later, her daughter called me.

"Sorry to bother you, but aside from telling you how much my mother appreciated your caring manner and your explanation of her macular problem, I just wanted to tell you that she really complains about her reading ability much more than she told you. She reads constantly during the day on her favorite chair and at night in her bed. She goes to bed at about eight thirty after dinner and often reads for hours. Reading is her life! She reads almost two books a week and keeps saying that she needs more light. We have already changed the light bulbs when she reads, and that seems to have helped a bit, but she still has trouble. It slows her down, which frustrates her. I guess she didn't tell you because she wants to be strong. She hates to complain. She is very proud—proud to be in such good shape at her age."

"I'm so glad you told me. Now that I know this, I think that she should see someone in our department who can help her more than I can. Her name is Katie, and she is an optometrist who runs our low vision clinic. She is an expert at exactly what your mother needs. Can I make an appointment for her? She is right here in my office, so all you have to do is to come to the same place again. Can you do that?"

"Of course."

"How about next Tuesday at 2:00 PM?"

"Fine."

"And I'll be there as well to introduce you."

"Great! Thank you, and by the way, Mother really loved your mini tour and meeting your president. That was very kind of you to think of arranging that. She could have talked to him forever!"

"Well, I can tell you that he really enjoyed meeting your mother."

On the following Tuesday, both women showed up to meet Katie. After about an hour of testing, it was obvious that the patient had lost considerable overall light sensitivity in both eyes, not unusual for anyone in her seventies. This meant that she would need more light to achieve her best visual potential. Arrangements were made to have Katie come to her home so that she could help create the optimal environment for reading, using improved lights and possibly some optical aids such as magnifiers. We had learned that such home visits were often necessary with elderly patients. Just giving them the aids and telling them to increase the power of the light bulbs really was not enough.

And so after two home visits, Katie had the situation under control. She had refined the reading glasses prescription and given her a large frame for reading only. She had attached two strong industrial spotlights to each side of the bed's headboard and done the same for her armchair downstairs. Then she got two magnifiers that doubled the print size, one for each reading location. The magnifiers she preferred turned out to be rather ugly industrial visors from the Home Depot, with a single wide flip-down glass, such as a wood carver might use. She didn't care what it looked like, only that it did the trick. She was also given a ruler, which she could put under each line she was reading to prevent her from getting lost on the page. Katie spent about two hours with her as she practiced reading. She was elated and showed her appreciation with a few tears.

During the next two or three years, patient and daughter came to our office every four months to check if things had changed, which they basically did not. There was perhaps some further decrease in overall retinal sensitivity, but her macular degeneration was stable.

Then, one morning, I got a phone call from the daughter that her mother had died in her sleep. She found her in the morning, sitting up in bed, with a book on her knee, wearing her visor, with the ruler in her clenched fist. All the bright lights still on, she had died doing her favorite thing. The daughter then asked me if I would please be an honorary pallbearer at the funeral.

"You don't have to do anything like carrying the casket. It's just honorary. You'll be listed in the church program."

"First of all, please accept my condolences. And your offer is very, very nice, but why me?"

"Well, it's very simple. You, and of course, your assistant Katie, were the most important people in her life toward the end."

"Thank you for the honor. Of course, I'm happy to do it."

Six months later, I noticed that her daughter had made an appointment to see me. She was curious if her mother's eye condition was hereditary and if she had any early sign of macular degeneration. Her eye exam was entirely normal. As she was leaving, she had one additional question: "Do you remember, about three years ago, that your department got an anonymous donation of a million dollars to establish a research professorship?"

"Yes, of course, that was fantastic, but I've always wondered who gave it. How do you know about it?"

"That was from my mother, just after the first time she saw you."

www.ingramcontent.com/pod-product-compliance
Lightning Source LLC
Chambersburg PA
CBHW020632220526
45464CB00001B/123